Food for Today

Student Workbook

Janis P. Meek, M.S., CFCS
Former Family and Consumer Sciences Teacher
Warren County High School
Warrenton, North Carolina

Alice Orphanos Kopan, M.Ed., M.A., CFCS

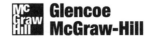

Glencoe McGraw-Hill

New York, New York   Columbus, Ohio   Woodland Hills, California   Peoria, Illinois

Editorial, design, and production assistance provided by
Howard Portnoy Editorial Services

Glencoe/McGraw-Hill

A Division of The **McGraw·Hill** Companies

Send all inquiries to:

Glencoe/McGraw-Hill
3008 W. Willow Knolls Drive
Peoria, Illinois 61614

ISBN 0-02-643051-7

Printed in the United States of America

5 6 7 8 9 10 066 04 03 02

TABLE OF CONTENTS

Unit Two ....Workspace, Tools, and Techniques

Chapter 12. Shopping for Food

Chapter 13. The Food Supply

Chapter 14. Buying for the Kitchen

Unit Four...................................Foods for Meals and Snacks

Chapter 15. Convenience Foods

Chapter 20. Food Combinations

Chapter 21. Baking

Unit Five...Expanding Your Horizons

Chapter 22. Foods of the World

Chapter 23. Foods of the U.S. and Canada

Chapter 24. Special Topics in Food

Chapter 25. Careers in Food and Nutrition

	Section 1-4

Activity

Food, Science, and Technology

Science and Technology to the Rescue

Directions: Today has been a day of problems for everyone in foods class. Fortunately, on the classroom bookshelf there are three books that might help class members solve their problems. Each book relates to a particular aspect of food science or technology.

Read each situation below. Then decide which of the books pictured would be most helpful in that situation. Write the call number of the appropriate book in the blank provided.

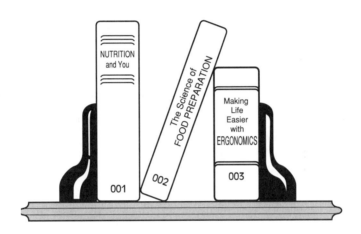

_____ 1. Tyrone didn't feel like doing anything today. He had slept late and skipped breakfast.

_____ 2. Teresa had a stiff neck from bending over the trash can to peel potatoes.

_____ 3. Callie complained because the group's menu had too much fat and contained foods from only two food groups.

_____ 4. The sink was too low for Devon, who is six feet one, so Laura had to wash the dishes.

_____ 5. Luther forgot to add the baking powder when he sifted the dry ingredients. The biscuits were hard and flat.

_____ 6. Theo's fruit salad looked unappealing because the bananas and apples turned dark.

_____ 7 Patrick dropped the pot of hot water because the handles were too small to grip.

_____ 8. Janine's pudding had a good taste, but the texture was very lumpy. She read the directions again to try to find out what she did wrong.

_____ 9. Frank could not figure out why the iced tea tasted bitter.

_____ 10. Beth got a blister on her hand when she tried to use the butcher knife to peel potatoes.

Activity

Choose to Make a Decision

Directions: Below are three situations. Choose one and identify the skill or skills from the box necessary to solve the problem. Then use the seven steps in the decision-making process to complete your solution.

Key Skills

directed thinking   communication   leadership   management

Situation 1
Your youth group is planning a cookout at the lake on Saturday night. You have been asked to plan the menu, which is for 20 people. You will have no electricity.

Skill(s): _____

_____

_____

Situation 2
Some classmates have decided to throw a surprise party for your teacher, who is retiring. Everyone has drawn a task from a slip of paper in a hat. You have drawn the task of baking a cake. You have never baked one before.

Skill(s): _____

_____

_____

Stuation 3
You and two friends are coming out of a movie and are looking for a place to go have a bite to eat. One friend suggests a restaurant that specializes in ribs, the other a fast-food restaurant. You have been concerned about nutrition and are short of cash right now.

Skill(s): _____

_____

Steps in Decision Making

1. Identify the decision to be made and your goals.

_____

_____

2. Consider your resources.

_____

_____

3. Identify your options.

_____

_____

4. Consider each option.

_____

_____

5. Choose the best option.

_____

_____

6. Carry out your decision.

_____

_____

7. Evaluate the result.

_____

_____

Study Guide

Directions: As you read Chapter 2, answer the following questions. Later you can use this study guide to review chapter information.

Section 2-1 The Role of Nutrients

1. What are vitamins? What function do they serve?

   _____

   _____

   _____

2. Why is water considered a nutrient?

   _____

3. Can malnutrition exist where food is abundant? Explain.

   _____

   _____

   _____

4. What are DRIs?

   _____

   _____

5. What are calories? How many calories are recommended for teen males, and active men and women?

   _____

   _____

   _____

Section 2-2 Carbohydrates, Fiber, and Proteins

6. How does your body respond if you don't eat enough carbohydrates? What is the consequence of this?

   _____

   _____

7. What kinds of foods contain fiber?

   _____

(Continued on next page)

Chapter 2 Study Guide (continued)

8. What are refined sugars? What two health problems are associated with them?

_____

_____

_____

9. What happens to excess protein in the body?

_____

10. How can you get all of the essential amino acids from plant food sources?

_____

_____

Section 2-3 Fats

11. Name two benefits that fats provide.

_____

_____

_____

_____

12. Identify two health risks associated with eating too much fat.

_____

_____

13. Identify the three basic kinds of fatty acids and tell the effect of each one on cholesterol levels.

_____

_____

_____

Section 2-4 Micronutrients

14. How does the body handle extra amounts of fat-soluble vitamins? What is the advantage of this?

_____

_____

_____

15. Identify two sources of vitamin D other than vitamin supplements.

_____

_____

_____

(Continued on next page)

16. Identify three types of minerals that your body needs.

_____

17. What are phytochemicals?

_____

_____

Section 2-5 How Your Body Uses Food

18. What is peristalsis?

_____

_____

_____

19. In what two ways does the stomach break down food?

_____

_____

20. Identity two basic ways your body uses energy.

_____

_____

Activity

You've Got a Case

Directions: You have been asked to fill in for a registered dietitian who works at a community health clinic. Below are notes about the dietitian's current caseload. Read the notes, and make recommendations using information from the section.

1. Ralph, age 38, is overweight. He spends much of his time watching television and snacking on brownies, nacho chips, and ice cream. He is not "in to" fruits or vegetables.

   Recommendations: _____

   _____

   _____

   _____

2. Marinda, age 8, was brought in by her mother. The mother does what she can to provide nutritious meals. Marinda, however, has always been a picky eater. She is not seriously underweight but does have bowed legs. The mother fears the child is suffering from malnutrition.

   Recommendations: _____

   _____

   _____

   _____

3. Celia, age 32, is pregnant with her first child. Lately, she has been feeling light-headed so much of the time that she has had to give up tennis and jogging. Upon questioning at the clinic, it was determined that Celia has put herself on an 800-calorie diet to make it easier for her to return to her normal weight after giving birth.

   Recommendations: _____

   _____

   _____

   _____

Activity

Nutrient Classifieds

Directions: This "Nutrient Classifieds" section of the newspaper contains want ads for specific forms of nutrients. In the space provided, write the name of the nutrient form described in each ad. Then list each nutrient form in the correct column below to show which type of nutrient it is. An example has been completed for you.

Nutrient Gazette
Classifieds

WANTED: Sucrose _____

    Form of sugar for use at the dining table

WANTED: _____

    Type of proteins found in plant sources

WANTED: _____

    Sugars removed from plants, processed, and used as sweeteners

WANTED: _____

    Type of proteins that supply all essential amino acids

WANTED: _____

    Complex carbohydrates found in dry beans and peas

WANTED: _____

    Form of sugar found in grains

WANTED: _____

    Plant material that absorbs water and contributes bulk

WANTED: _____

    Form of sugar found in milk

WANTED: _____

    Plant material that dissolves in water and may lower cholesterol

WANTED: _____

    Simple carbohydrates found naturally in fruits, grains, and milk

Carbohydrate	Fiber	Protein
Sucrose	_____	_____
_____	_____	_____
_____	_____	_____
_____	_____	_____

Section 2-3

Activity

Fats

Fats Fact Find

Directions: In each situation described, find the error in the person's reasoning. Then explain why the person's reasoning is incorrect.

1. When she discovered that her cholesterol was high, Merrille decided to stop eating fats entirely. "Who needs them?" she says. "The only thing they do is raise your cholesterol level."

Error(s):_____

_____

Explanation:

_____

_____

_____

_____

2. Gina is caring for her aunt who is on a low-cholesterol diet. Gina is careful to avoid serving her aunt green leafy vegetables, which she read somewhere contain hidden high amounts of cholesterol. She also uses low-fat milk when preparing her aunt's favorite dish, fluffy scrambled eggs.

Error(s):_____

_____

Explanation:

_____

_____

_____

_____

3. Trevor carefully checks the labels on the foods he buys. If a product contains even a gram of saturated fat, he will avoid buying it. However, Trevor reaches freely for products that contain the "healthy" fats—mono- and polyunsaturated.

Error(s):_____

_____

Explanation:

_____

_____

_____

Activity

Nutrition in the News

Directions: Below is the cover page of a newsletter titled Micronutrients Weekly. Read the story leads, filling in the blank in each headline. Select your answers from the list on the left of the page with the heading "In This issue..."

Micronutrient WEEKLY
Voume 6, Number 55

In This Issue. . .

- Anemia
- Beta Carotene
- Electrolytes
- Fat-Soluble
- Fortified
- Hemoglobin
- Major Minerals
- Osteoporosis
- Trace Minerals
- Water-Soluble

_____ : Deep, Dark Secret

The secret's out! This important phytochemical is found in deep yellow and dark green vegetables—the deeper, the darker, the better!

Outlook on _____

Scientists make no bones about it—lack of calcium can definitely cause bones to become weak and fragile.

_____ in Action

Potassium, sodium, and chloride keep body fluids in balance. What a great balancing act!

_____ Speak Up

Iron and copper speak up for the "silent minority" of minerals. Though small in number, they make a valuable contribution.

_____ Service

This substance will carry oxygen free of charge to all your body cells.

_____ Strikes Again!

Red blood cells are tired and weak. Lack of iron has reduced hemoglobin levels to an all-time low.

_____ Make It Big!

Calcium, phosphorus, and magnesium are in BIG demand. Large amounts are needed.

_____ Vitamins in Storage

Stores of vitamins A and D are in body fat and the liver. Call in orders as needed.

_____ Vitamin Down the Drain!

The vitamin C in a bushel of potatoes goes down the drain. Youth group dices, boils potatoes to make potato salad for a picnic.

Activity

Digestion at Work

Directions: Below is a cross section of a human digestive tract. Describe the task performed by each numbered organ on the corresponding line below.

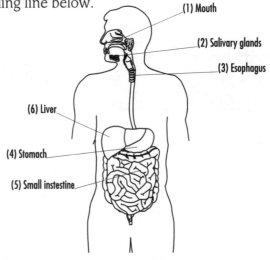

(1) Mouth

(2) Salivary glands

(3) Esophagus

(6) Liver

(4) Stomach

(5) Small instestine

1. _____

_____

2. _____

_____

3. _____

_____

_____

4. _____

_____

_____

5. _____

_____

_____

6. _____

_____

| Chapter 4 |

Study Guide

Planning Daily Food Choices

Directions: As you read Chapter 4, answer the following questions. Later you can use this study guide to review chapter information.

Section 4-1 Daily Meals and Snacks

1. What is an eating pattern?

_____

_____

2. Why is breakfast widely considered to be the most important meal of the day?

_____

_____

_____

3. Why is the midday meal important?

_____

_____

4. Why is snacking important during the teen years?

_____

_____

_____

5. What is grazing?

_____

_____

Section 4-2 Positive Eating Habits

6. What is appetite? What two types of influences shape a person's appetite?

_____

_____

7. What information should you include in a food record?

_____

_____

_____

(Continued on next page)

8. How do you go about reviewing a food record?

_____

_____

Section 4-3 Eating Out

9. What are the three main types of restaurants?

_____

10. Name four terms to avoid as a step toward controlling fat intake when eating in a restaurant.

_____

_____

11. Describe two methods for controlling portion size when eating out.

_____

_____

Section 4-4 The Vegetarian Lifestyle

12. In what important way is good vegetarian nutrition like good nutrition from any other eating pattern?

_____

13. What important nutrients are often missed in the vegan style of eating? How can vegans get these nutrients?

_____

_____

14. What foods can vegetarians substitute for foods from animal sources?

_____

15. Give three suggestions for vegans when eating out.

_____

_____

_____

Activity

What Do You Think?

Directions: Wendy's class is sponsoring a school-wide debate on the following topic: "Grazing is better for you than eating three traditional meals per day." Students have been asked to submit the following entry form stating their position (for or against the topic) and their arguments pro or con. Members of the debate teams will be drawn from the submitted entries. Fill in the entry form below to submit your ideas for the debate. Then you may want to organize your own class debate on this topic.

School-wide Debate!

Official Entry Form

Topic: "Grazing" is better for you than eating three traditional meals per day.

To enter: Fill out this entry form and return to Room _____.

Name: _____

Position (Circle the word that indicates whether you agree or disagree with the topic sentence):

FOR   **AGAINST**

Arguments: In the space that follows, explain why you are for or against the topic statement. Your arguments must be logical and clearly presented. Present your case as completely as you can on this form, because final debate contestants will be chosen on the basis of their responses.

_____

_____

_____

_____

_____

_____

_____

_____

_____

_____

_____

_____

_____

Activity

For the Record

Directions: An accurate food record is like a photograph. It tells a lot about a person's eating patterns. It can reveal both good and bad habits. The food record below belongs to a teen named Timothy. Study his food record and answer the questions on the next page.

Food Record

Saturday, January 12

Time	Food and Amount	Situation
10:30 A.M.	1 chocolate chip cookie 1 orange juice	slept late—skipped breakfast—went to mall
12:00 noon	1 slice pepperoni pan pizza 1 soft drink	ate at Pizza Palace in the mall
3:00 P.M.	1 plate of nachos, cheese 1 soft drink	ate a snack in the food court
5:30 P.M.	1/2 baked chicken breast 1 roll 1 glass iced tea 1 slice pecan pie	home for dinner—not very hungry—did not eat broccoli, rice, and pear salad
10:30 P.M.	1 cheeseburger 1 bag potato chips 1 soft drink	stopped at fast-food drive-through—ate on the way home

(Continued on next page)

Section 4-2 Activity (continued)

1. From which section of the Food Guide Pyramid do you see the greatest number of servings?

   _____

2. What foods did Timothy eat that fit in this category?

   _____

   _____

3. For which food group do you see no servings?

   _____

4. How many servings from that group should Timothy have eaten, according to the Food Guide Pyramid?

   _____

5. How could Timothy have changed his meals to include the recommended number of servings from this food group?

   _____

   _____

   _____

   _____

6. For better health what other changes would you advise Timothy to make in his food choices?

   _____

   _____

   _____

   _____

7. What facts do you learn about Timothy from his "Situation" column that may be influencing his eating habits?

   _____

   _____

   _____

   _____

Activity

Clues at the Corner Café

Directions: Read the menu for the Corner Café. Using the guidelines in your textbook, choose two nutritious meals you could order from the menu. Then answer the questions.

THE CORNER CAFÉ

APPETIZERS

Buffalo Wings $4.95
Tender chicken wings crisply fried

Fried Cheese $3.95
Mozzarella cheese breaded and deep fried; served with marinara sauce

Spicy Bean Soup $4.25
Made with black beans and fresh vegetables--delicious!

ENTREES

Pork Chops Deluxe $6.95
Two 4-ounce pork chops grilled over mesquite and topped with our special sauce

Fried Chicken $8.95
Succulent fried chicken served with corn on the cob and French fries

Sirloin Steak $12.95
12 ounces of top sirloin served with baked potato and steamed vegetables

Roasted Chicken $9.95
Seasoned with our special herbs, served with corn on the cob and baked potato

Baby Back Ribs $12.95
Slowly baked in barbecue sauce and served with beans and extra sauce

A LA CARTE

Sautéed Mushrooms $3.50
Baked Potato $1.95
Grilled Onions $2.95
French fries $1.95
House Salad $4.95
Caesar Salad $4.95

DESSERTS

Ice Cream Sandwich $3.95
Delicious vanilla ice cream between two layers of our homemade brownies; topped with hot fudge

Brownie $2.95
Made in our own kitchens; nuts, fudge, and all the trimmings

Fresh Fruit (Seasonal) $2.95
Ask your server which fruits are available

All-American Apple Pie $3.95
With ice cream $4.50

Frozen Yogurt $3.95

BEVERAGES

Iced Tea $0.95
Milk $1.50
Soft Drinks $1.50
Coffee $0.95

(Continued on next page)

Meal 1: _____

_____

_____

_____

_____

Meal 2: _____

_____

_____

_____

_____

Questions:

1. Suppose you were in the mood to eat pork chops. What could you do to ensure that they didn't come covered with a sauce high in fat?

   _____

   _____

   _____

   _____

2. Choose one of the entrées you did *not* list in this activity. Describe how you could lower the fat intake for that meal.

   _____

   _____

   _____

   _____

Activity

Menu "Before" and "After"

Directions: Almost any recipe can be adapted to the vegetarian lifestyle. To demonstrate this point for yourself, read the recipe on the left. On the right, rewrite the recipe, making appropriate substitutions for the type of vegetarian listed.

Recipe 1: Spicy Hominy

4 cups (1 L) beef broth, divided
2 oz. (60 mL) sliced mushrooms
4 cans hominy, drained
1 can cream-style corn
4 cans green chilies, drained
1 cup (250 mL) chopped green onions
2 tbsp. (30 mL) chili powder
2 cloves garlic
$^3/_4$ cup (190 mL) sour cream

Place 1 cup beef broth in Dutch oven; bring to a boil. Add mushrooms and remove from heat. Cover and let stand 10 minutes. Drain and chop mushrooms, reserving liquid. Pour reserved liquid through cheesecloth into bowl. Return liquid and mushrooms to pan. Stir in remaining ingredients. Bring to boil; cover, reduce heat, simmer 30 minutes, stirring occasionally. Spoon mixture into bowls and top with sour cream.

Recipe Modified for Ovo-Vegetarians

_____
_____
_____
_____
_____
_____
_____
_____
_____
_____
_____
_____
_____
_____

Recipe 2: Beef Vegetable Soup

1 cup (250 mL) chopped onion
3 cloves garlic
1 lb. (500 mg) beef, cubed and browned
1 small zucchini, sliced
1 can corn, drained
2 tomatoes, diced
1 cup (250 mL) beef broth
$^1/_2$ tsp. (3 mL) cumin
$^1/_2$ tsp. (3 mL) oregano

Sauté onion and garlic until brown; add remaining ingredients. Bring to boil; reduce heat, and simmer 20 minutes or until zucchini is tender.

Recipe Modified for Vegans

_____
_____
_____
_____
_____
_____
_____
_____
_____
_____
_____
_____
_____

● # Study Guide

Directions: As you read Chapter 5, answer the following questions. Later you can use this study guide to review chapter information.

Section 5-1 Maintaining a Healthful Weight

1. Explain why it is not realistic for most people to try to achieve an "ideal" body.

   _____

   _____

2. What is a healthy weight?

   _____

   _____

3. How is body mass index computed?

   _____

   _____

● 4. How can body fat tests help determine whether you should be worried about extra pounds?

   _____

   _____

Section 5-2 Weight Management

5. Why should teens be careful about following a weight-loss plan meant for adults?

   _____

   _____

   _____

6. Identify three disadvantages of poor weight-loss methods other than being potentially danger-ous to your health.

   _____

   _____

7. Identify the three general guidelines for successful weight loss.

   _____

   _____

   _____

●

(Continued on next page)

Chapter 5 Study Guide (continued)

8. Give three reasons why increasing your activity level is helpful in losing weight.

_____

_____

_____

9. Name two dangers of being underweight.

_____

_____

_____

Section 5-3 Keeping Active

10. Besides being useful in weight management what are two main benefits of keeping active?

_____

_____

11. What are the two main types of exercise?

_____

12. When selecting an activity program, what should you do to increase the likelihood of your sticking with the program?

_____

_____

Section 5-4 Nutrition for Sports and Fitness

13 Why is it important for athletes to eat plenty of carbohydrates?

_____

_____

14. Why are athletes advised to replace fluids during athletic events?

_____

_____

15. Identify two dangers of using anabolic steroids.

_____

_____

_____

Activity

"Weight"-ing Room

Directions: Your school has organized an advice clinic for students who think they have weight problems. Today is your day to volunteer in the clinic, under the supervision of the school nurse. Prescreen the following students by reading each one's complaint or question. Using what you know about healthy weight, tell what advice you would give in each case.

1. Evin is on the school wrestling team. While getting his yearly physical back in September, Evin recalls overhearing the nurse telling a patient with a BMI of 33 that he should lose some weight. Since then, Evin has discovered that his own BMI is 34. Evin believes he is at risk for serious health problems unless he sheds some pounds. What is your advice?

   _____

   _____

   _____

   _____

   _____

2. Geneva thinks she ought to lose weight. She is taller than most of the other girls in the school, and she weighs much more than most of them. She is active in several sports, and her waist-to-hip ratio is 0.75. What is your advice?

   _____

   _____

   _____

   _____

   _____

3. Randy has a typical "apple" shape. Although he occasionally joins in a neighborhood game of football, he doesn't like many sports; he prefers to work on his computer. Recently, Randy's parents have begun to suggest that he watch his weight. His waist-to-hip ratio is 0.99. What is your advice?

   _____

   _____

   _____

   _____

   _____

Activity

Weight Loss Winners and Losers

Directions: In the battle against weight, some people do lose—but not necessarily excess pounds. Some weight-loss programs and gimmicks can be costly both to the pocketbook and, more importantly, the individual's health. Read each portion of a media message for a weight-loss strategy below. Write "W" for each "winner" (a method based on sound health and nutrition principles). Write "L" for each "loser"—a method that poses a health risk or wastes consumers' money. If you write "L," use the space provided to explain the danger, risk, or form of loss that may occur.

_____ 1. Become one of thousands of satisfied users of the Pribble Plan, and watch the excess pounds melt away. Consume up to 750 calories a day on any foods you choose.

_____

_____

_____ 2. "Weight Zapper" pills contain a special secret ingredient that is sure to provide instant weight-loss success. Best of all, you can obtain "Weight Zapper" right over the counter at your pharmacy. No need for an expensive or time-consuming visit to your doctor for a prescription.

_____

_____

_____

_____ 3. At the Gilroy Clinic we use no fads or gimmicks. Pounds are lost gradually, using state-of-the-art behavior modification techniques.

_____

_____

_____ 4. Did you know eating liver can help you lose weight fast? That's the news from researchers at the University of Bellyville. In a soon-to-be-published report, the researchers claim that eating a pound of liver each morning can cause dramatic weight-loss results.

_____

_____

_____ 5. According to a new study at the Beltmore College of Physicians, walking—even at a leisurely pace—can help you maintain your weight, so long as the activity becomes a life-long habit.

_____

_____

Activity

The Exercise Connection

Directions: Imagine that you work for The Exercise Connection—a consulting and training firm that helps individuals choose physical activities that are right for them. The following are profiles of several of the company's clients. Read each profile. Then use information from the textbook to make recommendations for each client, along with reasons for your recommendations.

1. Client's name: Herb
   Age: 45
   Occupation: Accountant
   Hobbies/interests: Watching TV, dining at restaurants
   Remarks: Herb is 10 pounds overweight. He has expressed an interest in weight lifting.

   Recommendations: _____

   _____

   _____

   _____

2. Client's name: Celine
   Age: 32
   Occupation: Real estate agent
   Hobbies/interests: Reading about nature, participates in several local fund-raising organizations, PTA president, hot line volunteer
   Remarks: Celine has said she might like to join a volleyball team.

   Recommendations: _____

   _____

   _____

   _____

3. Client's name: Dallas
   Age: 29
   Occupation: Assistant Sales Manager
   Hobbies/interests: Attending football games
   Remarks: Dallas is a real "people" person and regrets having to travel approximately 20 weeks a year for work. His doctor has advised that he take up an activity that works the heart. He would like to combine his love of sports with his need for activity, perhaps by playing soccer.

   Recommendations: _____

   _____

   _____

Activity

Training Now and Then

Directions: The following is part of a book on nutrition advice for athletes as it might have appeared 30 or 40 years ago. Some of the statements contradict information in the textbook. Draw a line through each numbered sentence that is incorrect. Then write the correct information on the lines below with the same number as the incorrect sentence.

(1) During vigorous and extended periods of physical activity, the body's energy needs are greater than normal. (2) The most important thing for any athlete to remember, therefore, is to consume large quantities of foods high in proteins—such as steaks and chops—both during training and leading up to a competition. (3) It is protein, after all, that helps the body build muscles. (4) Short of this requirement, athletes have no nutritional needs beyond those of the average person.

(5) Turning to the matter not of what to eat but when to eat, in my long years as a coach and trainer, I have witnessed the ill effects of eating immediately before game time. (6) I disagree with numerous of my colleagues, who recommend consuming a full meal immediately before a contest. (7) A meal at this time is likely to disrupt the digestive process and compete with the muscles for energy. (8) I am, therefore, of a mind to counsel athletes to fast for a minimum of eight hours prior to game time.

(9) Finally, on the question of hydration, I am of the mind that consumption of liquids during athletic competition can place an undue strain on the bladder and other vital organs: I, thus, advise against drinking water during a game. (10) Instead, I strongly recommend that athletes consume salt tablets, to make up for sodium lost through perspiration.

(1) _____
(2) _____
_____
(3) _____
_____
(4) _____
_____
(5) _____
(6) _____
_____
(7) _____
_____
(8) _____
_____
(9) _____
_____
(10) _____

Study Guide

Directions: As you read Chapter 6, answer the following questions. Later you can use this study guide to review chapter information.

Section 6-1 Food and the Life Span

1. What is the life span? What are the five developmental stages of life?

_____

_____

2. Why should concern about good nutrition begin before pregnancy?

_____

_____

3. State four recommendations for the kinds and amounts of food to be eaten by expectant mothers.

_____

_____

_____

_____

_____

_____

_____

_____

4. At what stage of development should the first solid food be given? Which types of foods should be given, and why?

_____

_____

5. What special challenges do aging adults often face in meeting their nutritional needs?

_____

_____

_____

Section 6-2 Managing Health Conditions

6. Describe two ways in which stress can affect nutrition.

_____

_____

(Continued on next page)

7. Name two guidelines when helping care for someone who is ill or recovering from an illness.

_____

_____

_____

_____

_____

8. Which groups of people benefit from taking dietary supplements?

_____

_____

9. List four conditions that can require a special medically prescribed eating plan.

_____

_____

Section 6-3 Eating Disorders

10. What is an eating disorder?

_____

11. Identify three ways in which anorexics will try to lose as much weight as possible.

_____

_____

12. What is a binge eating disorder?

_____

_____

13. Why might it be harder to spot a person with bulimia nervosa than one suffering from anorexia nervosa?

_____

_____

14. Identify three health problems associated with anorexia nervosa.

_____

_____

_____

15. Identify three warning signs of bulimia nervosa.

_____

_____

_____

Activity

What the Doctor Ordered

Directions: Dr. Bullock, who specializes in nutrition for all ages, is working on a series of pamphlets containing sound eating advice to hand out to his patients. Unfortunately, his notes have become jumbled. Help the doctor sort out the mess. Write the number found next to each of Dr. Bullock's nutrition notes on the cover of the pamphlet in which it belongs. Some pieces of advice belong in more than one pamphlet. When you have finished, answer the questions on the next page.

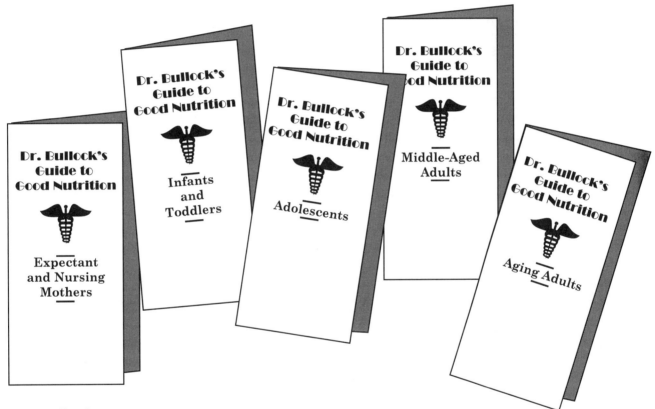

Dr. Bullock's Notes

1. . . . should have two daily servings of fish, poultry, meat, eggs, or dry beans.

2. . . . need increased amounts of foods that are rich in iron.

3. . . . as a result of which, they fail to get enough calcium or zinc.

4. . . . good choices include pieces of fruit (without skins), cheese, and crackers.

5. . . . need to drink eight glasses of water daily.

6. . . . need the same nutrients, though in smaller amounts.

7. . . . often don't get enough vitamin A in their eating plans.

8. . . . should choose a variety of low-fat, low-calorie foods.

9. . . . should eat plenty of citrus fruits and other foods that provide an abundance of vitamin C.

(Continued on next page)

Name _____ Date _____ Class _____

Questions

1. Which pamphlet would contain advice about dealing with food jags?

   _____

2. In which pamphlet should readers expect to find information about prenatal nutrient needs? Which readers of this pamphlet will learn that they can look forward to gaining as much as 35 to 45 pounds (16 to 20 kg)?

   _____

   _____

3. Mrs. Larsen, one of Dr. Bullock's patients, just turned 75 and is on a limited income. What problems regarding the nutrient needs of people in her situation do you think she might learn about in Dr. Bullock's "Aging Adults" pamphlet? What steps might she take to correct these problems?

   _____

   _____

   _____

   _____

Activity

A Day with the Boswicks

Directions: Meet the Boswicks. The story that follows describes a typical morning in the Boswick household. Read the story. Then, on the lines provided, identify the problems with the family's eating habits, and suggest healthful changes.

Mr. Boswick stood at the range, stirring a pot of oatmeal. "Breakfast!" he called out to his family.

Jeb Boswick, the Boswicks' teenage son, was the first to reach the kitchen. "Sorry, Dad," Jeb said as he pulled the collar of his jacket upward and grabbed his book bag. "I've got a big test this morning. I'm too fired up to eat."

"Make that two of us," said Mrs. Boswick. "I'm late for work." She grabbed a bottle on the kitchen counter labeled "all-purpose mineral supplement," popped a pill in her mouth, and washed it down with a gulp of orange juice. "At least I look after my nutritional needs," she said pointedly, looking straight at Jeb, who was halfway out the door. Jeb shrugged, stomped over to the toaster, picked up a piece of toast, and stuffed the whole thing into his mouth. He slammed the door behind him.

"Kids!" Mrs. Boswick said, shaking her head. "Bye, dear." She kissed Mr. Boswick on the cheek and headed out to the garage.

Mr. Boswick turned off the flame under the pot and stared at the uneaten pot of oatmeal. He had just begun spooning some into a bowl when he heard a sneeze behind him. He turned to find his 11-year-old daughter Kim standing behind him. "Young lady," he scolded, "what are you doing out of bed?"

Kim sneezed again and said, "All the noise down here woke me up."

Mr. Boswick felt her forehead. "You're burning up, Kim. You get back into bed, and I'll bring you a tray."

"I don't feel like eating anything," she replied, sniffling.

"You're the boss, honey," her father said. He carried his bowl of oatmeal over to the kitchen table where the morning paper was waiting.

"Dad," Kim said. "You're not going to eat that—are you?"

"And why shouldn't I?" he asked.

"You know—what the doctor said about your diabetes acting up."

"Don't you worry about me, honey," he replied with a smile. "I'm not putting any milk or butter on my oatmeal."

_____
_____
_____
_____
_____
_____
_____

Activity

The HELP Line

Directions: Imagine that you are a volunteer for a community help line geared to helping people with health-related problems. Below are several calls that have come in this afternoon. Answer each call in your own words, using information from the textbook.

Caller 1: Hi, my name is Delia. I'm 16. My problem is that I'm just plain too fat! I've tried everything I can to lose weight—laxatives, strenuous exercise, starvation diets—but nothing helps. My friends all tell me I already look plenty skinny, but I know they're just being nice. What can I do to lose weight?

Your Response:

_____

_____

_____

_____

_____

Caller 2: I'm worried about my daughter. Every evening after dinner, she leaves the table to go to the bathroom. Then she comes back, smiling, to help with the dinner dishes. The pattern is always the same. Recently, while cleaning her bathroom, I found some laxatives. Do you suppose my daughter has an ulcer or something?

Your Response:

_____

_____

_____

_____

_____

Caller 3: Hello, HELP line? I'm calling because I think I have an eating disorder. I love to eat, especially burgers and fries. I also get sore throats a lot, and I hear that that's a sign of an eating disorder. Do you think I ought to see a doctor?

Your Response:

_____

_____

_____

_____

_____

Activity

"Clean Up Your Act!"

Directions: Read each situation. Then use the spaces provided to list all examples of unsafe food handling practices. You should find at least four problems in the first act and at least five in the second act.

It's Saturday. The Brody house is the scene of unexpected chaos and calamity. Mom and Dad are both sick in bed. Fifteen-year-old Denise is away at camp. That leaves eight-year-old twins Tammy and Tommy to take charge. Let's take a look as the drama unfolds.

Act 1: Breakfast

Tammy and Tommy woke up hungry at 7:00 AM. After using the bathroom, they both headed straight for the kitchen to get breakfast. After rinsing out four cereal bowls in the sink and wiping them with a dish towel, Tammy reached for the cereal and filled the bowls. When she had to sneeze unexpectedly, she turned her head and covered her mouth with her hand. Then she reached for spoons and napkins. Tommy went to the refrigerator to get the milk. He spilled only a few drops on the counter, which he wiped up with the dish towel. After eating his own cereal, Tommy took a breakfast tray to Mom and Dad. Tammy stayed in the kitchen to clean up.

_____

_____

_____

_____

_____

_____

_____

_____

_____

_____

_____

_____

_____

_____

(Continued on next page)

Section 7-3 Activity (continued)

Act 2: Lunch

    It's time for lunch. Tommy gets out bologna and sliced cheese, while Tammy grabs a loaf of bread and a jar of mayonnaise. Tommy arranged four slices of bologna on the counter and topped one each with cheese. Tammy spread mayonnaise on eight slices of bread and put the sandwiches together. When Rover scratched on the back door, Tommy let him in while Tammy moved the sand-wiches aside to make room for Rover's dish. Tommy fixed Rover's Gravy Chunks while Tammy poured milk and got out chips. Tommy wiped the counter clean where Rover's dish and the sand-wiches had been. Lunch tasted great! Afterwards, the twins left the dishes neatly stacked in the sink. Tammy said she would wash them later. Before heading outdoors to play, Tammy removed a package of chicken from the freezer and put it on the counter to thaw for that night's dinner.

_____

_____

_____

_____

_____

_____

_____

_____

_____

_____

_____

_____

_____

_____

_____

_____

_____

_____

_____

_____

_____

_____

Activity

A Measure of Success

Directions: You will be able to measure ingredients successfully if you know the appropriate measuring tools to use for each ingredient. Imagine that you have the measuring tools listed below. Using only these tools, describe how you would measure the following amounts of ingredients.

Tools Available:

Measuring spoon set: $\frac{1}{4}$ tsp., $\frac{1}{2}$ tsp., 1 tsp., 1 Tbsp.
Dry measures: $\frac{1}{4}$ cup, $\frac{1}{3}$ cup, $\frac{1}{2}$ cup, 1 cup

How would you measure ...

1. $\frac{3}{4}$ cup of sugar

   _____

   _____

2. $\frac{2}{3}$ cup of fine bread crumbs

   _____

   _____

3. $\frac{3}{4}$ teaspoon vanilla extract

   _____

   _____

4. $1\frac{1}{4}$ tablespoons of cornstarch

   _____

   _____

5. $3\frac{1}{4}$ cups of flour

   _____

   _____

6. $\frac{5}{8}$ cup of cornmeal

   _____

   _____

7. $\frac{7}{16}$ cup of sugar

   _____

   _____

8. $\frac{3}{8}$ tsp. pepper

   _____

   _____

Activity

Decreasing Recipe Yield

Directions: In the left column are listed the ingredients for two recipes that yield 6 servings. In the right column, rewrite the ingredient lists to decrease the yield as specified.

Decrease to 2 servings:

1 lb. lean boneless beef sirloin steak _____

2 tsp. peeled, minced ginger root _____

3/4 tsp. grated tangerine rind _____

1/2 cup fresh tangerine juice _____

2 Tbsp. low-sodium soy sauce _____

1 1/2 tsp. cornstarch _____

1/2 pound fresh snow pea pods _____

1 tsp. dark sesame oil _____

1 cup fresh bean sprouts _____

3/4 cup diagonally sliced celery _____

3 cups cooked long-grain rice _____

Decrease to 3 servings:

2/3 cups yellow cornmeal _____

1/3 cup all-purpose flour _____

3/4 tsp. baking powder _____

1/4 tsp. baking soda _____

1 tsp. sugar _____

1/4 tsp. dried crushed red pepper _____

3/4 cup nonfat buttermilk _____

2 1/2 Tbsp. frozen egg substitute, thawed _____

1 Tbsp. margarine, melted _____

Activity

The Task at Hand

Directions: On the line after each task listed below, write the name of the tool that should be used to complete the task. Be specific. For example, if a knife should be used, tell what kind of knife. If more than one tool can be used for the task, list all of the possibilities.

1. Mixing dry ingredients: _____

_____

2. Trimming fat from meat and meat from bones: _____

_____

3. Whipping cream: _____

_____

4. Folding blueberries into muffin batter: _____

_____

5. Draining the water from cooked vegetables: _____

_____

6. Stirring to keep food from sticking to the pan while cooking: _____

_____

7. Chopping vegetables: _____

_____

8. Mixing, combining, and blending: _____

_____

9. Pureeing vegetables for a soup: _____

_____

10. Peeling thin-skinned fruits: _____

_____

Activity

Team Plan

Directions: Plan a team time schedule for a 4-member lab group to prepare and serve pizza snacks with orange juice. Lab begins at 10:45 and ends at 11:35. Review the recipe and work plan on pages on pages 252-253 in the text. Then use the form below to develop your team plan. Use check marks to indicate which person should do each task.

Time	Task	Person			
		1	2	3	4
10:45	Get ready	✓	✓	✓	✓
10:53	Split English muffins				
10:53	Prepare to wash dishes				
10:53	Wash vegetables				
10:53	Assemble equipment				
10:55	Chop onions and peppers				
10:55	Slice mushrooms				
10:55	Shred cheese				
10:55	Wash tools as used				
11:02	Assemble pizzas				
11:05	Broil pizzas				
11:11	Prepare to serve				
11:11	Pour orange juice				
11:12	Serve				
11:13	Eat				
11:23	Clear table				
11:23	Wash counters				
11:23	Wash dishes				
11:23	Dry, put away dishes				
11:27	Dispose of garbage				
End of Lab					

	Chapter 9
Study Guide	**Cooking Methods**

Directions: As you read Chapter 9, answer the following questions. Later you can use this study guide to review chapter information.

Section 9-1 Equipment for Cooking

1. Identify the three major parts of a range.

   _____

   _____

2. What are the two major fuel sources for most ranges?

   _____

3. What may happen if the air flow in a gas range is blocked?

   _____

   _____

4. Name the two main types of electric range heating units.

   _____

   _____

5. How is energy produced in a microwave oven?

   _____

   _____

   _____

6. Name five types of cookware.

   _____

   _____

   _____

7. What is the best way to remove baked-on food from bakeware?

   _____

   _____

Section 9-2 Heat and Cooking

8. Name the three types of energy transfer central to all cooking.

   _____

   _____

(Continued on next page)

9. Identify three changes in food that result from the application of heat.

_____

_____

10. Name three specific nutrients that can be destroyed by heat.

_____

_____

Section 9-3 Conventional Cooking Techniques

11. Identify one advantage and one disadvantage of steaming foods.

_____

_____

12. Explain why foods cook faster in a pressure cooker than with other methods.

_____

_____

13. What is preheating?

_____

_____

14. To what foods is broiling well-suited?

_____

_____

15. What two cooking methods are combined in braising? In stir-frying?

_____

_____

Section 9-4 Microwave Cooking Techniques

16. What is a watt?

_____

17. Which foods are most successfully cooked in a microwave oven?

_____

_____

18. How do concentrations of sugar and fat affect how a food cooks in a microwave oven? What problem can this create?

_____

_____

_____

(Continued on next page)

19. List four factors besides composition that affect how a food cooks in a microwave oven.

_____

_____

20. Why should you avoid using products containing recycled paper in a microwave oven?

_____

_____

21. Give two tips for arranging foods in a microwave oven.

_____

_____

_____

_____

22. What is standing time?

_____

_____

23. What is the best way to adapt a standard recipe for the microwave oven?

_____

24. Besides the usual recipe features, what information should a microwave recipe contain?

_____

_____

_____

25. What happens if dirt builds up inside a microwave oven?

_____

_____

Activity

Cook's Choice

Directions: Chuck Wiley and his family are buying new appliances and cookware for their newly remodeled kitchen. However, the family members cannot agree on what to buy. Their arguments for and against each item are shown below. Evaluate their arguments and make your own recommendation for what they should buy in each case. Point out any false reasoning that you find. You may recommend one of the items they mention, or you may suggest something entirely different that might better suit their needs.

1. Mrs. Wiley wants a gas range because she wants immediate control over the heat levels on the burners. Mr. Wiley wants an electric range because he doesn't want to have to keep lighting the pilot light on a gas range.

   _____
   _____
   _____
   _____
   _____

2. Chuck thinks they ought to buy both a toaster and a toaster oven. He often fixes his own breakfast early in the morning, and he thinks toast from the toaster tastes better. He wants a toaster oven to warm up small amounts of other foods. Mr. Wiley says they can't have both because they would take up too much counter space.

   _____
   _____
   _____
   _____
   _____

3. Jessie and Julie often make baked goods to sell at various club events. The family has agreed to let them choose the bakeware. Julie wants to buy metal bakeware with a nonstick finish to make cleanup easier. Jessie wants to buy glass bakeware because it is easier to use than metal.

   _____
   _____
   _____
   _____
   _____

Activity

The Heat Is On

Directions: The box below contains three descriptions of the effects of heat on food. Read the descriptions, then answer the questions that follow.

A. After reading his mother's instructions, Pete removed the pot of soup from the refrigerator and placed it on the burner, stirring the soup from the bottom up to the top. When Pete tasted the soup moments later, Pete was surprised to find it was still cold. Only the part nearest the bottom of the pot gave off the slightest trace of warmth.

B. The lost hikers returned to camp exhausted by the scorching sun; their hunting expedition had been a failure. To their surprise, the supply of berries they had picked and left on the flat rock were hot to the touch, and some had split open and lay in puddles of purple juice.

C. On contact with the hot grill, the steaks began to sizzle and sputter; flames leaped up around the edges. Soon, Jill turned the first steak over. A delightful aroma of meat and bar-becue-scented smoke filled the air. The steak was branded with brown-black stripes where it had been in contact with the red-hot grate.

1. Which of the descriptions involves radiation? Explain your answer.

   _____

   _____

2. What of the three methods of heat transfer is suggested by the manner in which Pete stirred the soup? Is this method of heat transfer limited to cooking on the top of the range?

   _____

   _____

3. What method of heat transfer has cooked the steak? How do you know?

   _____

   _____

4. In which of these methods are nutrients being lost? Explain.

   _____

   _____

   _____

5. Which of the heat sources described is the least efficient? Why?

   _____

   _____

   _____

Activity

Conventional Cooking Techniques

Getting a Handle on Cooking Techniques

Directions: Matt had all the recipes on his computer filed in terms of cooking method. When his hard drive "crashed," he lost a lot of important data. Help Matt reorganize his computer files. Decide in which folder on Matt's computer each partial recipe belongs. Write the folder name in the space following the recipe. NOTE: Each folder name can be used only once.

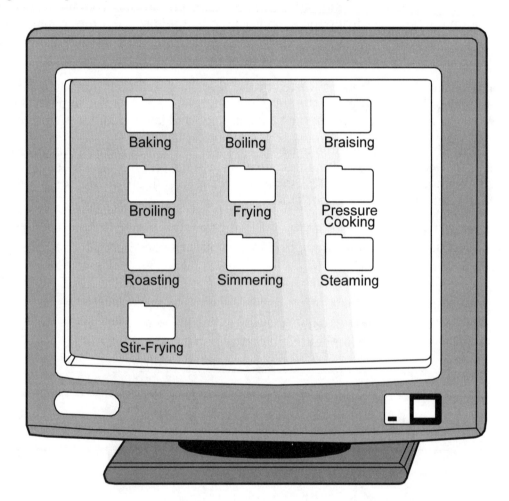

1. Place the filled muffin pans in a preheated oven.

   Cooking Technique: _____

2. Carefully lower the contents of each egg into the boiling salted water; poach gently until done.

   Cooking Technique: _____

3. Melt 2 tablespoons of butter, and add the chopped onion. Cook until the onion turns golden.

   Cooking Technique: _____

(Continued on next page)

4. Remove the bay leaf from the sauce, turn up the heat, and cook vigorously until the sauce has reduced by one-third and is quite thick.

   Cooking Technique: _____

5. Place the duck uncovered on a rack in a shallow pan. Periodically baste the bird with the fat that has dripped into the pan.

   Cooking Technique: _____

6. If you don't have a specially made basket, place the peas in a fine-mesh strainer and insert in the saucepan above the boiling water. Cover and cook until the peas are tender.

   Cooking Technique: _____

7. Transfer the browned stew meat, vegetables, and broth into the pot. Follow the manufacturer's instructions.

   Cooking Technique: _____

8. When the oil in the wok has begun to "dance," add the ginger, garlic, chopped onion, and celery. Move the ingredients around in the oil to coat them. Add the chicken pieces and stir again.

   Cooking Technique: _____

9. Place the turkey burgers on the grid; cook three inches from the heat source for about 7 minutes, or until the tops of the burgers are quite brown.

   Cooking Technique: _____

10. Place the browned beef roast back into the Dutch oven. Add the carrots and potatoes. Add enough broth or water to half-cover the roast. Cover the pan and cook over low heat for about 2 hours, or until meat is fork-tender.

    Cooking Technique: _____

Questions

11. Suppose Matt wanted to create new folders for his computer labeled "Dry-Heat Methods." Which of the recipes described earlier would fit in this category? Which would fit in a folder labeled "Combination Methods"?

    _____

    _____

    _____

12. Which of the recipes could be prepared using another cooking method? Explain.

    _____

    _____

13. Matt recently found tempting-sounding recipes for doughnuts and navy bean soup. In which file folder would each belong?

    _____

    _____

Activity

Microwave Mishaps

Directions: Microwave ovens have become very popular lately in Range City. However, several of the 50 people who have bought microwaves in the last two weeks have had trouble with them. Read each person's problem. In the space provided, explain what went wrong and what the person should do differently next time.

1. Once a week after school, Rochelle uses the microwave oven in the school lunchroom to pop popcorn for the other people on the cheerleading squad. When she tries to pop the same popcorn in her family's new microwave at home, the popcorn burns, even though she uses exactly the same settings.

   _____

   _____

   _____

   _____

   _____

2. Everyone in Renie's family has a different schedule, so the family makes up nutritious dinners ahead of time and stores them in the freezer. Renie loves the new microwave oven—it takes only 6 minutes on the high setting to cook a frozen meal. Today, her friend Amy is eating dinner with her. She puts two frozen dinners in the microwave and cooks them for 6 minutes, but at the end of the cooking time they're just barely warm.

   _____

   _____

   _____

   _____

   _____

3. Kevin's first experience with his microwave oven was a disaster! First, he carefully washed a baking potato and cooked it on the high setting for 6 minutes. During that time, he went into the basement to get the boneless chicken breast out of the freezer. When he came back to the kitchen, he discovered that the potato had exploded! "Oh, well," he thought, "at least I'll have some chicken for dinner." After cleaning up the potato mess, he cooked the chicken until it tested done. Then he let it stand for 10 minutes. The chicken was tough and hard to chew.

   _____

   _____

   _____

   _____

   _____

Study Guide

Directions: As you read Chapter 10, answer the following questions. Later you can use this study guide to review chapter information.

Section 10-1   Serving Family Meals

1. Why are family meals important?

   _____

   _____

   _____

2. What can happen when people read or watch television while they eat?

   _____

   _____

   _____

3. What is a place setting?

   _____

   _____

4. What is a cover?

   _____

   _____

5. How is flatware arranged in a cover?

   _____

   _____

   _____

6. Identify two advantages of plate service.

   _____

   _____

   _____

7. Where in the cover are rolls placed in formal meals? In less formal meals?

   _____

   _____

   _____

(Continued on next page)

Section 10-2   Mealtime Etiquette

8. What is table etiquette?

_____

_____

9. In what way can good table manners be an asset in the working world?

_____

_____

10. When may you reach for serving dishes?

_____

_____

11. How should you handle coughing or sneezing at the table?

_____

_____

_____

12. What information should you include when making reservations?

_____

_____

13. What should you do if you find a mistake on the check for a meal?

_____

_____

14. What is a gratuity? What is another name for a gratuity?

_____

_____

15. What should you do if you voice a complaint to your server about a meal, and nothing is done?

_____

_____

Activity

Recipe for an Enjoyable Meal

Directions: Read the paragraph about meals in the Andares household. On the lines below, list the problems the Andares have at mealtime and describe a way to correct each problem.

Meals are very informal at the Andares home. Everyone's schedule is different, so the family rarely eats together. In the interest of sharing family time together, Mr. Andares occasionally calls for everyone to be present at the dinner table. On these occasions, dinner is a "thrown-together" affair. No one takes the time to decorate the table or even set it properly. Everyone is usually cranky after a long day of working. The older children resent not being able to play basketball or visit their friends. The younger children constantly bicker at the table. The television is usually on, because Mr. and Mrs. Andares like to watch the evening news. Carla dislikes family dinners because it is her job to clean up the kitchen, and when the whole family eats at once, there's a huge mess to clean up.

_____

_____

_____

_____

_____

_____

_____

_____

_____

_____

_____

_____

_____

_____

_____

_____

_____

_____

Activity

Dear Hemley

Directions: You are filling in for Hemley, the advice columnist for your local newspaper, while he is on vacation. Below are several letters you have received requesting advice. Answer each letter in the space provided.

1. Dear Hemley,

   After my cousin's wedding dinner, my sister and I got into a fight over whether you're supposed to wait until everybody is served before you start eating. I say you should eat before the food gets cold. Who's right?

   —Linda

   Dear Linda:

   _____

   _____

   _____

   _____

   _____

2. Dear Hemley,

   My family recently went to this expensive restaurant to celebrate my grand-mother's birthday. You won't believe what we saw. There was a man at a near-by table eating the olives on his plate—using his fingers! You should spread the news that it's impolite to eat with the fingers.

   —Ray

   Dear Ray

   _____

   _____

   _____

3. Dear Hemley,

   After we won the regionals, our school chess club went out to a nice restau-rant as a victory party. When the check came, we were charged for an extra beverage. The club president, said the thing to do was to take it out of the serv-er's tip. When I said we should point it out to the server, everybody else laughed and rolled their eyes. Did I make a fool out of myself?

   —Rosalita

   Dear Rosalita:

   _____

   _____

   _____

Chapter 11

Study Guide

Planning Meals

Directions: As you read Chapter 11, answer the following questions. Later you can use this study guide to review chapter information.

Section 11-1 Basic Meal Planning

1. Identify three factors to consider when planning a meal.

   _____

   _____

2. List four resources related to meal planning.

   _____

   _____

3. Explain two things to think about when considering food choices and availability.

   _____

   _____

4. What are the five characteristics of meal appeal?

   _____

5. Identify three advantages of planning meals for a week or more at a time.

   _____

   _____

   _____

   _____

Section 11-2 Challenges in Meal Planning

6. What is the first step to finding time for home-prepared meals?

   _____

7. Give two suggestions for preparing flexible meals.

   _____

   _____

8. Describe a common dilemma singles face in shopping and preparing meals.

   _____

   _____

(Continued on next page)

Chapter 11 Study Guide (continued)

9. What are two suggestions for dealing with last-minute changes in meal plans?

_____

_____

Section 11-3   Food Costs and Budgeting

10. What is a budget?

_____

_____

11. What percentage of family income does the average middle-income family spend on food?

_____

12. List four factors that affect food expenditures.

_____

_____

_____

_____

13. Describe the steps in setting up a food budget.

_____

_____

_____

_____

14. If find you can't seem to stick to your food budget, what are your two options?

_____

_____

_____

15. Identify four sources of help from people who cannot afford to buy enough food.

_____

_____

_____

Activity

Resource Tradeoffs

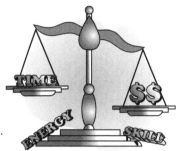

Directions: Few people are able to plan and create meals without trading off resources in one way or another. Read the examples below. Suggest at least one tradeoff that would help each person or family eat more nutritiously. Write your answers on the lines below each example.

1. Katarina says her family doesn't have time to eat nutritiously. Her mother is working full-time and going to school at night. Her father has an evening job, so he sleeps in the daytime and is away during the dinner hour. Katarina's school and athletic activities keep her busy until about 6:00 each evening.

   _____

   _____

   _____

   _____

   _____

2. Len loves to cook, and he's good at it, but his family has recently had to pay enormous medical bills for his father. Len's father's health forced him to quit his job, and Len's mother has to stay home to take care of his father. Money is scarce and his father's appetite isn't very good. The doctor encourages the family to fix tempting dishes for him; there are no dietary restrictions.

   _____

   _____

   _____

   _____

3. Everyone in Tina's family enjoys cooking. However, the family doesn't have much money, and they have only basic kitchen tools. They can't afford many of the small, specialized appliances that some families have.

   _____

   _____

   _____

   _____

   _____

Activity

Challenges

Directions: The situations below involve challenges in meal planning. Read each situation. Using what you have learned about meal planning, give one suggestion to help each person meet the challenge.

1. Fran's husband left home for 6 months of basic military training. Fran has become frustrated trying to cook dinner for one. She has to throw away food every night.

   _____

   _____

   _____

   _____

   _____

2. When Kathy arrived home, she found that her husband was already there with two friends he had brought home for dinner.

   _____

   _____

   _____

   _____

   _____

3. Everyone in the Abbot house is always on the run. No one seems to have time to cook. All are very tired of deli foods and eating out.

   _____

   _____

   _____

   _____

   _____

4. William loves to cook, but has time to cook only on weekends. During the week, he gets very tired of eating out.

   _____

   _____

   _____

   _____

   _____

Name _____ Date _____ Class _____

Activity

Food Costs and Budgeting

Food Spending Record

Directions: Review the food spending record below. Then answer the questions on the next page.

Money Spent for Food						
April 7-13						
Su	M	Tu	W	Th	F	Sa
Breakfast from drive-through: $3.25		Morning snack from convenience mart: $1.75				Breakfast out: $4.50
	Lunch in cafeteria: $2.50	Lunch in cafeteria: $2.50	Lunch in cafeteria: $2.50	Lunch in cafeteria: $2.50	Lunch in cafeteria: $2.50	Lunch in food court: $4.25
Snack from vending machine: $1.00		Pick up groceries at convenience mart: $12.50	Take-out dinner: $7.50	Groceries from supermarket: $54.00	Dinner out: $12.75	Groceries from convenience mart: $17.75
April 14-20						
Su	M	Tu	W	Th	F	Sa
Lunch out: $8.00	Lunch in cafeteria: $2.50	Lunch in cafeteria: $2.50	Lunch in cafeteria: $2.50	Lunch in cafeteria: $2.50	Lunch in cafeteria: $2.50	
	Dinner from deli: $5.50	Groceries from supermarket: $22.00	Afternoon snack at service station: $2.00	Pick up groceries at convenience mart: $13.50	Snack from vending machine: $1.50	Dinner out: $16.75

(Continued on next page)

Section 11-3 Activity (continued)

Questions

1. What was the total amount of money spent for food during the first week? _____

2. What was the total amount of money spent for food during the second week? _____

3. What was the average amount spent per week? _____

4. What percentage of the total money spent for food during the first week was spent for eating out? (Include everything except groceries.) _____

5. List suggestions which could help this person to reduce spending for food.

   _____

   _____

   _____

   _____

   _____

   _____

   _____

	Chapter 12
# Study Guide	**Shopping for Food**

Directions: As you read Chapter 12, answer the following questions. Later you can use this study guide to review chapter information.

Section 12-1   Before You Shop

1. How do cooperatives keep food prices low?

   _____

   _____

2. Identify two advantages and two disadvantages of shopping at convenience stores.

   _____

   _____

3. What should you consider when choosing a place to shop?

   _____

   _____

4. When should you avoid shopping for food?

   _____

   _____

5. What is impulse buying?

   _____

   _____

6. What are staples?

   _____

   _____

7. Name and briefly describe the two types of coupons.

   _____

   _____

   _____

   _____

(Continued on next page)

Section 12-2 Food Labels

8. What two types of information about calories are included on "Nutrition Facts" panels on food products?

_____

_____

9. What do the terms "reduced" or "fewer" mean on a food label?

_____

_____

10. What does the phrase "good source of" refer to on a food label?

_____

_____

11. What information is given in code dating? Why is this important?

_____

_____

12. What purpose is served by the UPC on products?

_____

_____

_____

_____

Section 12-3 In the Supermarket

13. Name four supermarket departments.

_____

_____

14. Identify three methods used in comparison shopping.

_____

_____

15. List three do's and don'ts of courteous shopping.

_____

_____

_____

Activity

Plan of Action

Directions: You are helping to buy the groceries for your school's annual awards banquet. The main ingredients for the recipes to be used are listed below. You will need to buy enough of each ingredient to feed 30 people. Using this information, figure out how much of each ingredient you need and create an organized shopping list to help you shop efficiently.

Spicy Grilled Chicken
½ cup lime juice
1½ Tbsp. minced jalapeño pepper
6 (6-ounce) skinned chicken breast halves
Yield: 6 servings

Frozen Dessert
1 envelope unflavored gelatin
2 (8-ounce) packages frozen raspberries
1 (6-ounce) can frozen lemonade concentrate
1 cup fat-free milk
⅓ cup sugar
Yield: 10 servings

Tossed Salad
3 Tbsp. orange juice
2 Tbsp. balsamic vinegar
2½ cups torn leaf lettuce
1 cup sliced fresh strawberries
2 Tbsp. green onions, thinly sliced
1 Tbsp. sesame seeds, toasted
Yield:6 servings

	Item	Amount Needed for Recipe
Produce		
Meat, Poultry, Fish		
Dairy		
Shelf-Stable Foods		
Frozen Foods		

Activity

Label Lingo

Directions: Below is a Nutrition Facts panel for processed American cheese slices. Use the information from the textbook and the panel to answer the questions that follow.

Nutrition Facts
Serving Size 1 slice (21g)
Servings per Package 16

Amount Per Serving

Calories 70   Calories from Fat 46

% Daily Value*

Total Fat 5g	**8%**
Saturated Fat 3.5g	**17%**
Polyunsaturated Fat 1.5g	
Cholesterol 15mg	**5%**
Sodium 330mg	**14%**
Total Carbohydrate 2g	**1%**
Dietary Fiber 0g	
Sugars 1g	
Protein 4g	

Vitamin A 4%	•	Vitamin C 0%
Calcium 10%	•	Iron 0%

1. What is the size of one serving of this product? How many servings total are there in the package?

   _____

2. What percentage of the Daily Value for sodium does this product provide?

   _____

3. What percentage of the product's calories come from fat? Explain how you arrived at this answer.

   _____

   _____

(Continued on next page)

Name _____ Date _____ Class _____

Section 12-2 Activity (continued)

4. Which micronutrients are provided in a single slice of cheese? What DV of each does the food provide?

_____

5. Imagine that a person made a sandwich containing two slices of this cheese and one slice of bologna. If the slice of bologna provided 26 percent of the person's DV for saturated fat, what percentage of the person's daily fat intake would be provided by the two different sandwich fillings combined?

_____

6. Do you think the food label on which this Nutrition Facts panel appears might contain the word "low"? Why or why not?

_____

_____

_____

_____

7. Compare this Nutrition Facts panel with one for a comparable product in your school foods lab, at home, or in a local supermarket. Which of the two products represents a more healthful choice? Explain your answer.

_____

_____

Activity

A Supermarket Report Card

Directions: As noted in the textbook, supermarkets can vary in terms of setup and even the types and nature of nutritional information they offer. How does your local supermarket stack up? Find out by taking the checklist below to a popular store in your community—ideally the one where you or your family shops. Complete the information. (1 is lowest; 5 is highest.) Then assign the store a grade, noting what changes you might recommend to the management.

Store Name: _____
Address: _____

✔   Times when the store is most/least crowded: _____
✔   Day(s) on which coupons are offered: _____
✔   Rating of departments in terms of cleanliness (circle one):
    Produce   1 2 3 4 5
    Meat, poultry, and fish   1 2 3 4 5
    Refrigerated foods   1 2 3 4 5
    Frozen foods   1 2 3 4 5
    Other: _____   1 2 3 4 5
✔   Rating of departments in terms of quality of merchandise (circle one):
    Produce   1 2 3 4 5
    Meat, poultry, and fish   1 2 3 4 5
    Refrigerated foods   1 2 3 4 5
    Frozen foods   1 2 3 4 5
    Other: _____   1 2 3 4 5
✔   Problem areas in store (e.g., poor ventilation): _____
    _____
✔   Helpfulness and courtesy of staff (circle one):   1 2 3 4 5
✔   Helpfulness and courtesy of management (circle one):   1 2 3 4 5
✔   Quality of store/generic brands (circle one):   1 2 3 4 5
✔   General level of courtesy among customers (circle one): 1 2 3 4 5
✔   Special, hard-to-find items the store carries: _____
    _____
✔   Remarks: _____
    _____
    _____

Grade: _____
What recommendations might you make to the store manager on ways that the store could improve its service to customers?

_____
_____

Study Guide

Directions: As you read Chapter 13, answer the following questions. Later you can use this study guide to review chapter information.

Section 13-1 Where Does Food Come From?

1. How does hydroponic farming differ from traditional farming?

   _____

   _____

2. Identify four commercial preservation methods.

   _____

   _____

3. Describe modified atmosphere packaging and its effect on food.

   _____

   _____

   _____

4. What is the role of distributors in the food supply network?

   _____

   _____

   _____

5. How much of every dollar spent on food goes to the farmer? Where does the rest go?

   _____

   _____

   _____

Section 13-2 A Safe Food Supply

6. What is the EPA? What is its role in regulating food safety?

   _____

   _____

   _____

7. How does the FDA respond when it believes a food is unsafe?

   _____

   _____

   _____

(Continued on next page)

8. What does GRAS stand for? What does it mean when an additive is on the GRAS list?

_____

_____

9. Why are some experts critical of fat substitutes in general? Of Olestra in particular?

_____

_____

_____

_____

10. Identify two concerns associated with irradiation.

_____

_____

11. Tell what contaminants are and give two examples.

_____

_____

Section 13-3 The Global Food Supply

12. What is one problem with feeding grain to food-producing animals?

_____

_____

13. How do poor roads in developing countries contribute to famine?

_____

_____

14. How is food used as a political weapon?

_____

_____

15. Identify three groups or agencies that teach farmers in developing countries how to increase food production.

_____

_____

Activity

From Farm to Table

Directions: The familiar foods pictured below are all staples of the American table. Use the pictures and information from the textbook to answer the questions that begin at the bottom of this page and continue on to the next.

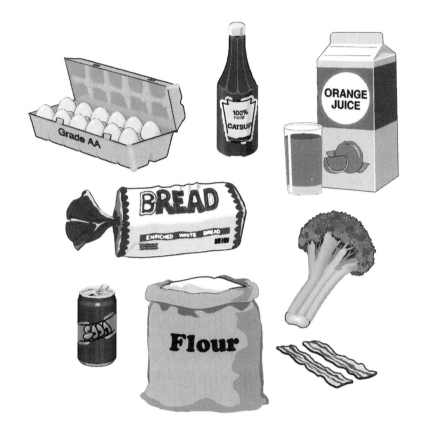

1. Which of the foods shown underwent the simplest processing? Explain your answer.

   _____

   _____

2. Which of the foods do you think underwent the most processing? Explain your answer.

   _____

   _____

   _____

(Continued on next page)

Section 13-1 Activity (continued)

3. Which of the foods shown is available in aseptic packages? By what other name is this packaging known?

_____

4. Which of the foods shown underwent the process of curing?

_____

5. Which of the foods were derived from other foods? From which foods did they come?

_____

_____

6. Which of the foods may have been a product of hydroponic technology?

_____

7. Which of the foods would you be least likely to encounter in a supermarket in the packaging shown?

_____

_____

8. Which of the items shown is most likely to be affected in price by natural disasters? Which is most likely to be affected in price by consumer damage?

_____

_____

_____

_____

9. Which of the foods is able to trace its origin in some fashion to a farm? Explain.

_____

_____

_____

_____

Activity

On the Other Hand

Directions: Below are newspaper headlines that describe the benefits or evils of using a particular food additive. Each of the stories suggested by the headline has another side to it. In the space following each headline, write a headline of your own, encapsulating the opposite view of the additive in question.

1. CLASS ACTION SUIT FILED AGAINST FOOD MANUFACTURER; COMMUNITY CLAIMS IRRADIATION CAUSED CANCER OUTBREAK

   Your headline: _____

   _____

2. STATE REPORTS INCREASE IN AFLATOXIN LEVELS OVER PREVIOUS FOUR YEARS

   Your headline: _____

   _____

3. FDA APPROVES FAT SUBSTITUTE FOR COMMERCIAL USE

   Your headline: _____

   _____

4. FOOD SCIENTISTS DEVELOP NEW, HARDIER STRAIN OF TOMATO

   Your headline: _____

   _____

5. STUDY LINKS SACCHARIN TO CANCER IN LAB RATS

   Your headline: _____

   _____

6. "MY FAMILY WAS POISONED BY CHEMICAL RESIDUES," CLAIMS BLAIRTON MOM

   Your headline: _____

   _____

Activity

Hope for the Hungry

Directions: Read the description of Erbordia—a fictional country that has many of the same problems real developing countries have. In the space below the description, list problems that affect the country's food supply. Then create a plan to eliminate as many of the problems as possible.

Times are hard in Erbordia. Most of the people survive by farming the land they rent from the rich landowners who run the country's political activities. The rent is high, and some of the people have begun to revolt. In return, the landowners have begun withholding food supplies from various areas. The crops are small, but the people don't know how to increase the yield. To make matters worse, this year's harvest has been almost completely wiped out by a mysterious disease that attacks the crops. Famine and disease are widespread.

Problems in Erbordia:

_____
_____
_____
_____
_____
_____
_____
_____

Plan for Helping Erbordia:

_____
_____
_____
_____
_____
_____
_____
_____
_____
_____
_____

Study Guide

Directions: As you read Chapter 14, answer the following questions. Later you can use this study guide to review chapter information.

Section 14-1 Consumer Skills

1. What is the principal of a loan?

   _____

2. Explain what interest on a loan is and how it is expressed.

   _____

   _____

3. What is indicated by an Underwriters Laboratories seal on electrical appliances?

   _____

   _____

4. Identify two problems with service contracts.

   _____

   _____

   _____

5. Describe two things you should do when you get a new appliance home.

   _____

   _____

   _____

   _____

Section 14-2 Choosing Kitchen Equipment

6. List three types of cooktops besides traditional gas burners and electric coils.

   _____

   _____

7. Identify three feature options of microwave ovens.

   _____

   _____

   _____

(Continued on next page)

8. List three conditions that kitchen tools should meet to be considered wise purchases.

_____

_____

_____

_____

9. List four materials that may be used for everyday tableware.

_____

_____

Section 14-3 Designing a Kitchen

10. Identify four questions regarding users' lifestyle that should asked when planning a kitchen.

_____

_____

_____

_____

11. What problems do work triangles sometimes present for today's kitchens?

_____

_____

12. Describe an efficiency problem that may arise in corridor kitchens.

_____

_____

13. Identify three storage aids that can be added to existing cabinets.

_____

_____

_____

14. What is grounding? Why is it important?

_____

_____

15. What is life-span design?

_____

_____

_____

_____

Activity

Calculating Payments

Directions: Most people need to buy appliances on credit at one time or another. Understanding how to calculate interest and total payments can help you keep track of how much you owe at any point. This activity will help you learn to calculate these important figures.

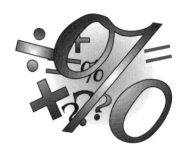

Here's an example that will help you understand the process: Anita purchases a refrigerator-freezer for $1,195. She buys it on credit at an interest rate of 12%, and she will pay off the loan in 24 equal monthly payments.

The total amount she will pay (including interest) is:

purchase price + (12% of purchase price)

To calculate 12% of the purchase price, you have to change the 12% into a decimal by dividing it by 100:

$$12 \div 100 = 0.12$$

Now use the formula:

$$\$1,195 + (0.12 \times \$1,195) = \$1,338.40$$

So Anita will pay a total of $1,338.40 for the refrigerator-freezer.

Next Anita needs to determine how much will each monthly payment will be. To find that amount, simply divide the total amount she will pay by the number of payments she will make:

$$\$1,338.40 \div 24 = \$55.76666,$$
which when rounded = $55.77

How much will Anita still owe on the refrigerator-freezer after she has made 14 payments? To find out, multiply her monthly payment by 14, and then subtract that answer from the total amount she will pay:

$$\$55.77 \times 14 = \$780.78$$

$$\$1,338.40 - \$780.78 = \$557.62$$

(Continued on next page)

Section 14-1 Activity (continued)

Now it's your turn. For each of the following, find the total amount owed (including interest), the amount of each monthly payment, and the amount still owed after the stated number of payments are made. Refer to the example on the previous page if necessary.

1. David uses credit to buy a range for $445. The interest rate is 11%, and he will make 12 monthly payments.

   Total amount owed: _____

   Amount of each monthly payment:_____

   Amount still owed after he makes 7 payments: _____

2. Sol buys a $640 dishwasher on credit. The interest rate is 14%, and he will make 18 monthly payments.

   Total amount owed: _____

   Amount of each monthly payment:_____

   Amount still owed after he makes 9 payments: _____

3. Athena buys a freezer for $985. The interest rate is 12%, and she will make 36 monthly payments.

   Total amount owed: _____

   Amount of each monthly payment:_____

   Amount still owed after she makes 23 payments: _____

4. Martin buys a deluxe microwave oven for $524. The interest rate is 10%, and he will make 12 monthly payments.

   Total amount owed: _____

   Amount of each monthly payment:_____

   Amount still owed after he makes 4 payments: _____

5. Yolanda buys a washer and dryer for a combined price of $880. The interest rate is 13%, and she will make 15 monthly payments.

   Total amount owed: _____

   Amount of each monthly payment:_____

   Amount still owed after she makes 11 payments:_____

Name _____ Date _____ Class _____

Activity

Choosing Appliances Wisely

Directions: You are choosing appliances for your new, all-electric apartment. You have decided to buy a range, refrigerator-freezer, and dishwasher, and you have narrowed the choices to the items listed below. All of the products are UL- approved and have good warranties and come from reputable dealers. Look at the floor plan of the kitchen and study the choices. Then write your final choice for each appliance. Explain your reasons.

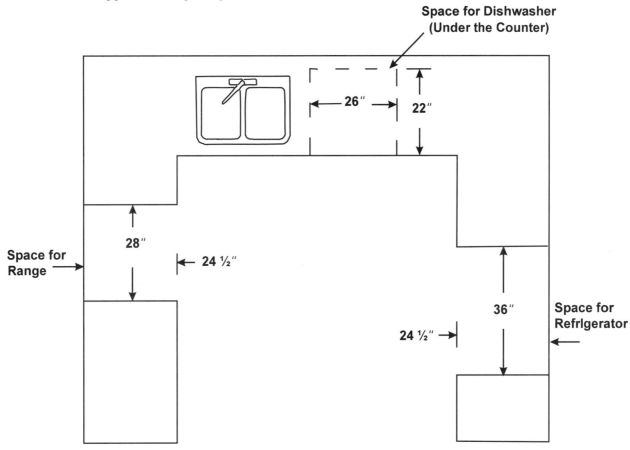

Remember: The width of the appliances must be slightly smaller than the openings in the cabinets for the appliances to fit correctly.

Choices for Range

Model A: 25"deep, 27" wide; has continuous-cleaning oven, traditional electric coils; controls are on raised panel at back of range. Cost: $637.

Model B: 24½" deep, 28½" wide; has self-cleaning oven, smooth cooktop; controls are on front center of range and are easy to read. Cost: $750.

Model C: 24½" deep, 27" wide; has self-cleaning oven, sealed gas burners; controls are easy to reach from front of range. Cost: $549.

Model D: 24½" deep, 27" wide; basic convection oven with traditional electric coils; controls are at front of range, but are hard to read. Cost: $575.

(Continued on next page)

Section 14-2 Activity (continued)

Choices for Refrigerator-Freezer

Model A: 25" deep, 35" wide; hinged on left, separate temperature controls, automatic icemaker, self-defrosting. Cost: $945.

Model B: 25" deep, 36" wide; hinged on right, single temperature control, no icemaker, self-defrosting. Cost: $849.

Model C: 26" deep, 34" wide; hinged on left, separate temperature controls, no icemaker, self-defrosting. Cost: $895.

Model D: 25" deep, 35" wide; hinged on right, separate temperature controls, no icemaker, manual defrost. Cost: $799.

Choices for Dishwasher

Model A: 23" deep, 25" wide; adjustable racks; 4 cycle settings, including energy-saving setting; runs quietly. Cost: $625.

Model B: 21" deep, 25" wide; adjustable racks; 3 cycle settings, including energy-saving setting; runs quietly. Cost: $595.

Model C: 21" deep, 25" wide; non-adjustable racks; 3 cycle settings, no energy-saving setting, no information about noise level. Cost: $415.

Model D: 21" deep, 26" wide; adjustable racks, 4 cycle settings, including energy-saving setting, no information about noise level. Cost: $659.

Your Final Choices

Range: _____

Reasons (include reasons you chose not to buy the other models):

_____

_____

_____

_____

Refrigerator-Freezer: _____

Reasons (include reasons you chose not to buy the other models):

_____

_____

_____

_____

Dishwasher: _____

Reasons (include reasons you chose not to buy the other models):

_____

_____

_____

_____

Section 14-3

Activity

Designing a Kitchen

How Far?

Directions: Review Cheryl's steps as she prepares breakfast. As you read each item in the list below, use a pencil to trace Cheryl's path in the kitchen. Assuming that each tile on the floor represents one step, write down the number of steps needed for each task. Add up the number of steps Cheryl takes. Then answer the questions on the next page.

Note: Assume that when Cheryl goes to the range, she stops in front of the center of the range; when she goes to the refrigerator, she stops in front of the center of the refrigerator, and so on.

Cheryl went to the kitchen to prepare an omelet and orange juice. She began at the sink, where she washed her hands. Then she went:

1. to the refrigerator to get eggs, cheese, margarine, and milk.

2. to the countertop beside the range to put down ingredients.

3. to the drawer to the left of the sink to get a fork and an egg turner.

4. to the base cabinet on the right side of the sink to get a mixing bowl.

5. to the countertop beside the range to beat eggs and milk.

6. to the base cabinet beside the range to get a skillet.

7. to the range to melt margarine and cook the omelet.

8. to the wall cabinet to the right of the sink to get a plate.

9. to the drawer left of the sink to get a flat grater.

10. to the drawer beside the refrigerator to get waxed paper on which to grate cheese.

11. to the countertop beside the range to grate the cheese.

12. to the range to add the cheese and to complete cooking the omelet.

13. to the trash can under the sink to dispose of waxed paper.

14. to the wall cabinet to the right of the sink to get a glass.

15. to the refrigerator to get the orange juice.

16. to the sink to deposit soiled utensils.

17. to the range to get the omelet.

U-Shaped kitchen

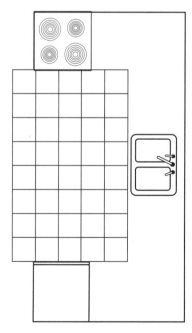

No. of steps: _____

(Continued on next page)

Section 14-3 Activity (continued)

1. What is the importance of saving steps in the kitchen?

   _____

   _____

2. How might Cheryl save steps by storing items differently in her kitchen?

   _____

   _____

   _____

   _____

3. How might Cheryl save steps by changing her kitchen work habits?

   _____

   _____

   _____

   _____

4. Suppose you are a kitchen designer. Cheryl is thinking of remodeling her kitchen and has asked you for suggestions. What changes, if any, would you make in the floor plan of her kitchen? Why? (Use the space at the bottom of the page to draw a sketch of your ideas, if needed.)

   _____

   _____

   _____

   _____

(Continued on next page)

Study Guide

Directions: As you read Chapter 15, answer the following questions. Later you can use this study guide to review chapter information.

Section 15-1 Choosing Convenience Foods

1. What is a convenience food?

   _____

2. Name two kinds of manufactured foods.

   _____

3. Identify the nutritional advantages of eating foods made from TSP.

   _____

   _____

4. What is a formed product?

   _____

   _____

5. Why are convenience foods costly?

   _____

   _____

6. Why are convenience foods potentially problematic from a nutritional standpoint?

   _____

   _____

7. Name three steps consumers can take to offset the high cost and nutritional limitations of convenience foods.

   _____

   _____

Section 15-2 Cooking with Convenience

8. Describe two ways of increasing the nutrient value of dry mixes used to make main or side dishes.

   _____

   _____

9. List four common types of convenience foods.

   _____

(Continued on next page)

Chapter 15 Study Guide (continued)

10. What does reconstitute mean?

_____

_____

11. Identify three advantages of making your own convenience foods.

_____

_____

_____

_____

12. Name three general types of homemade convenience foods.

_____

_____

13. Give three examples of pre-prepared ingredients.

_____

_____

14. Describe two ways of "cooking for the freezer."

_____

_____

15. What is the secret to a successful homemade mix?

_____

_____

Activity

Weighing the Pros and Cons

Directions: As noted in the textbook, using convenience foods has both its advantages and disadvantages. Some of each are identified below. Read the situations below and on the next page. In the space below each situation, write the advantage (Advantage P) or disadvantage (Disadvantage N) each describes. The first one has been done for you.

Advantages
P—Provides for special dietary needs
R—Reduces preparation time for meals
O—Offers greater variety of foods with less space and equipment
S—Saves time and energy

Disadvantages
C— Cost is usually high
O—Often high in sodium, sugar, and fat
N—Not always as nutritious as nonconvenience foods
S—Sometimes short on flavor

1. Steve buys nonfat dry milk because he has very little space in his tiny refrigerator.

   _____

2. Annette has stopped buying "Sweet-Crunch" cereal since she read the label and noticed the product contains three different kinds of sweeteners.

   _____

3. Roy has been buying an egg substitute called "Good-Eggs" since he had his cholesterol level checked.

   _____

4. Cathy has never liked instant mashed potatoes. She says they just aren't as good as the home-made kind.

   _____

(Continued on next page)

Section 15-1 Activity (continued)

5. Sherrika has noticed an increase in food spending since she started working. She has been buying more frozen dinners and quick foods.

_____

6. Jim cannot understand why anyone would want to make a cake from scratch. With very little time and effort, he can have a cake mix prepared and in the oven.

_____

7. Grandmother is not as energetic as she once was. She now buys frozen yeast dough to make hot rolls for family dinners.

_____

8. Ward was surprised to learn that the frozen vegetables he bought had fewer vitamins than fresh forms.

_____

9. The newlyweds bought "Waffle-o's," which could be warmed in the toaster. They do not own a waffle iron.

_____

10. Ingrid buys refrigerated flour tortillas when she makes her family's favorite enchilada dish. Since the recipe takes three hours to prepare, she appreciates all the shortcuts she can find.

_____

Activity

Rhyme or Reason

Directions: Listed below are tips for cooking with convenience foods. These tips help to make the most of the pros and minimize the cons. Read each tip and think about why it is a good suggestion. Use the space provided to write either a rhyme or a reason that explains the tip. The first one is done for you, with an example of both a rhyme and a reason.

Tip # 1   Use convenience foods in combination with fresh foods within a meal.
   Rhyme or Reason:
   (Rhyme) Mix quick and fresh foods upon your plate
   For meals that are healthful and taste really great.
   (Reason) Fresh foods offer nutrients and flavor to help make up for lost nutrients and
   flavor in convenience foods.

Tip # 2. Substitute fat-free milk or water for whole milk to prepare dry mixes.
   Rhyme or Reason:
   _____
   _____
   _____
   _____

Tip #3. Prepare quick-cooking grains as nutritious side dishes.
   Rhyme or Reason:
   _____
   _____
   _____
   _____

Tip #4. Use frozen dinners as "emergency" meals, not as routine main dishes.
   Rhyme or Reason:
   _____
   _____
   _____
   _____

(Continued on next page)

Section 15-2 Activity (continued)

Tip #5. Follow directions on convenience food packages exactly.
Rhyme or Reason:

_____

_____

_____

_____

Tip #6. Read the package each time you use a product.
Rhyme or Reason:

_____

_____

_____

_____

Tip #7. Follow directions for thawing as closely as directions for cooking.
Rhyme or Reason:

_____

_____

_____

_____

Tip #8. Follow "use by" dates on refrigerated convenience foods.
Rhyme or Reason:

_____

_____

_____

_____

Tip #9. Try variations suggested on packages.
Rhyme or Reason:

_____

_____

_____

_____

Tip #10. Make your own convenience foods.
Rhyme or Reason:

_____

_____

_____

_____

Study Guide

Directions: As you read Chapter 16, answer the following questions. Later you can use this study guide to review chapter information.

Section 16-1 Choosing Vegetables and Fruits

1. Name three antioxidants that vegetables and fruits provide.

   _____

   _____

2. What are tubers? Name an example.

   _____

   _____

3. Why are seeds high in carbohydrates and other nutrients?

   _____

   _____

4. Explain how to ripen fruits after buying them.

   _____

   _____

5. Where should potatoes, onions, and sweet potatoes be stored? Why?

   _____

   _____

6. How should most other fresh produce be stored?

   _____

   _____

Section 16-2 Preparing Raw Vegetables and Fruits

7. Why should you wash vegetables even if you are planning to peel them?

   _____

   _____

8. Why should you avoid soaking produce in water?

   _____

   _____

(Continued on next page)

9. What is enzymatic browning? How can it be prevented?

_____

_____

10. How should you store cut produce you don't plan to use immediately?

_____

_____

Section 16-3   Cooking Vegetables and Fruits

11. How does cooking affect the texture of vegetables and fruits?

_____

_____

12. What precaution should you take before microwaving whole vegetables that have a skin? Why?

_____

_____

13. In what way are potatoes especially convenient to bake?

_____

_____

14. Give two reasons for adding sugar to the water when poaching fruit.

_____

_____

15. Identify two advantages and one disadvantage of microwaving fruits.

_____

_____

Section 16-1

Activity

Choosing Vegetables and Fruits

Three of a Kind

Directions: From each group of four, select the one vegetable or fruit that does not belong with the other three and cross it out. Write the remaining "three of a kind" on the three cards. Label each threesome with the term in the Feature Box that identifies a trait they have in common.

Feature Box

- seasonal vegetables
- cruciferous vegetables
- seed vegetables
- available all year
- drupes

- tubers
- citrus fruits
- leafy vegetables
- bulb vegetables
- melons

- "fruit" vegetables
- tropical fruits
- root vegetables
- stored at room temperature

Example: broccoli   kale   on~~i~~ons   mustard greens

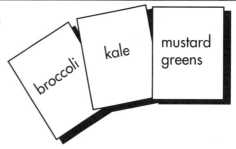

Common feature: _dark-green vegetables_

1. pineapples   pears   papayas   bananas

Common feature: _____

2. beets   carrots   asparagus   turnips

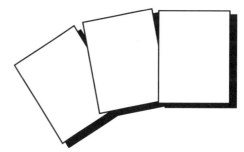

Common feature: _____

3. potatoes   yams   celery   sweet potatoes

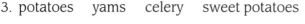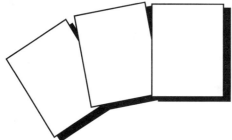

Common feature: _____

4. grapefruit   tangerines   oranges   apples

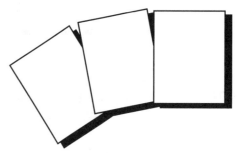

Common feature: _____

(Continued on next page)

◆ *Food For Today* **Student Workbook 117**

5. carambola   cherries   peaches   plums

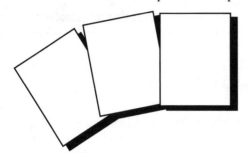

Common feature: _____

6. lettuce   spinach   kiwi   collards

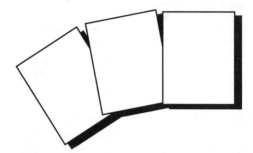

Common feature: _____

7. onions   garlic   carrots   scallions

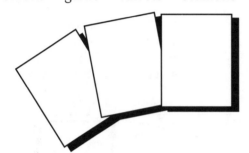

Common feature: _____

8. cantaloupe   casaba   iceberg   honeydew

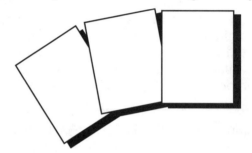

Common feature: _____

9. corn   beans   peas   radishes

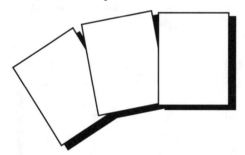

Common feature: _____

10. cucumbers   celery   eggplant   tomatoes

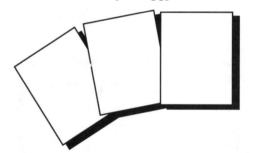

Common feature: _____

11. broccoli   cabbage   rutabagas   squash

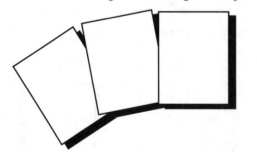

Common feature: _____

12. cabbage   onions   potatoes   yams

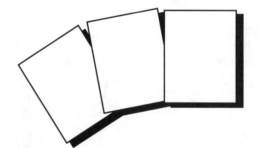

Common feature: _____

Activity

You've Got Some Explaining to Do

Directions:
Write an explanation for each of the following facts about preparing raw vegetables and fruits.

1. Wash vegetables and fruits even if you plan to peel them.

Explanation: _____

_____

_____

2. A brush is needed to wash potatoes thoroughly.

Explanation: _____

_____

_____

3. Avoid letting produce soak in water.

Explanation: _____

_____

_____

4. Although the edible skins on vegetables and fruits are a source of added nutrition and fiber, some people feel better paring them away.

Explanation: _____

_____

_____

5. Cut vegetables and fruits into the largest possible pieces.

Explanation: _____

_____

_____

6. When preparing a fruit salad, coat the cut pieces of banana, apple, pear, and other such fruits with a little lemon juice.

Explanation: _____

_____

_____

(Continued on next page)

Section 16-2 Activity (continued)

7. Arrange fresh vegetables and fruits artistically for serving.

Explanation: _____

_____

_____

8. Squeeze excess air out of sealed plastic bags containing fresh vegetables.

Explanation: _____

_____

_____

9. Serve cut vegetables and fruits as soon after cutting as possible.

Explanation: _____

_____

_____

10. Keeping cut-up vegetables in the refrigerator is a good idea.

Explanation: _____

_____

_____

Activity

Do You Know the Question?

Directions: Each item below is the answer to a specific question about cooking vegetables and fruits. Your job is to come up with a question for each. Write the question in the space provided. The first one has been done for you.

1. Serve cooked vegetables and fruits with the cooking liquid whenever possible.

Question: _What is one way of minimizing the loss of vitamin C and other nutrients when_ _cooking vegetables?_

2. The cell walls become softer and more tender.

Question: _____

_____

3. It provides the color of green vegetables.

Question: _____

_____

4. The flavors are released and made more noticeable.

Question: _____

_____

5. Fewer precious nutrients are lost because the vegetables are not cooked in water.

Question: _____

_____

6. These minerals react with sulfur compounds in vegetables, resulting in a loss of vitamin C, folic acid, and vitamin E.

Question: _____

_____

7. Arrange tender parts toward the center and less tender parts toward the edges.

Question: _____

_____

8. They are usually cut in half, the seeds removed, and the halves placed on a baking sheet.

Question: _____

_____

(Continued on next page)

Name _____ Date _____ Class _____

Section 16-3 Activity (continued)

9. This cooking method adds fat and calories to vegetables and should be used sparingly.

Question: _____

10. It helps the fruit maintain its sweetness and helps keep its shape during cooking.

Question: _____

11. Add lemon or orange rind, a cinnamon stick, or vanilla.

Question: _____

12. Unlike poaching, the goal of the method is to helps breaks down the texture of the fruit.

Question: _____

13. Firm fruits—such as apples, pears, and bananas—give the best results.

Question: _____

14. Fruits keep their fresh flavor and their shape.

Question: _____

15. Like vegetables, they may burst unless you take care to puncture them with a fork in several places, as you would do with vegetables, before cooking them so that they don't burst.

Question: _____

Study Guide

Directions: As you read Chapter 17, answer the following questions. Later you can use this study guide to review chapter information.

Section 17-1   Choosing Grains and Grain Products

1. What are grains?

   _____

   _____

2. What are the three main parts of every grain seed, or kernel?

   _____

   _____

   _____

3. What is converted rice?

   _____

   _____

4. In what ways are cornmeal and grits similar? What is the difference between them?

   _____

   _____

5. Why might you add wheat germ to foods?

   _____

   _____

6. Are wheat bread and whole wheat bread the same product? Explain.

   _____

   _____

   _____

7. Identify three guidelines for storing grains and grain products.

   _____

   _____

   _____

   _____

   _____

(Continued on next page)

Section 17-2 Preparing Grains and Grain Products

8. How would you prepare bulgur?

   _____

   _____

9. What is the approximate cooked yield of one cup (250 mL) of barley? Of kasha?

   _____

   _____

10. How can you keep cooked pasta hot?

    _____

    _____

11. Explain how to prepare leftover cooked pasta for freezing.

    _____

    _____

Section 17-3 Legumes, Nuts, and Seeds

12. What are legumes?

    _____

    _____

13. How do legumes and grains work together to provide protein in an eating plan?

    _____

    _____

14. Briefly describe how to soak beans.

    _____

    _____

15. List four types of edible seeds.

    _____

    _____

Activity

Grains of Truth

Directions: Read carefully each statement about grains and grain products. Place a check mark in the blank for each true statement. For each untrue statement, write a corrected statement on the line provided. You should have to replace only one word in each untrue statement to make it true.

_____ 1. Grains are the most important staple in the world food supply.

_____

_____ 2. Grains are stems of plants in the grass family.

_____

_____ 3. The germ is a tiny embryo that will grow into a new plant.

_____

_____ 4. The outer protective coat found on a seed of grain is the bran.

_____

_____ 5. The bran is the food supply for the embryo.

_____

_____ 6. Complex carbohydrates are found in the germ of grains.

_____

_____ 7. During processing of grain, the outer husk is removed to leave the kernel, or grain seed.

_____

_____ 8. The entire kernel is used in enriched grain products.

_____

_____ 9. When 10 percent of the daily value of a nutrient is added to a grain product, the product is said to be fortified.

_____

_____ 10. Long-grain rice tends to be very moist and sticky when cooked.

_____

_____ 11. The whole-grain form of rice is brown rice.

_____

_____ 12. Couscous is a popular grain in the Middle East.

_____

(Continued on next page)

Section 17-1 Activity (continued)

_____ 13. Tortillas are an example of a Mexican grain product.

_____

_____ 14. The coarsely ground endosperm of corn is called bulgur.

_____

_____ 15. Triticale is a cross between wheat and rye.

_____

_____ 16. Ground bran cereals are high in fiber content.

_____

_____ 17. Wheat germ is added to other foods for more nutritional value.

_____

_____ 18. Pasta is made from a flour and water dough.

_____

_____ 19. Pita bread is a type of leavened bread.

_____

_____ 20. Cooked grains should be placed in the refrigerator for long-term storage.

_____

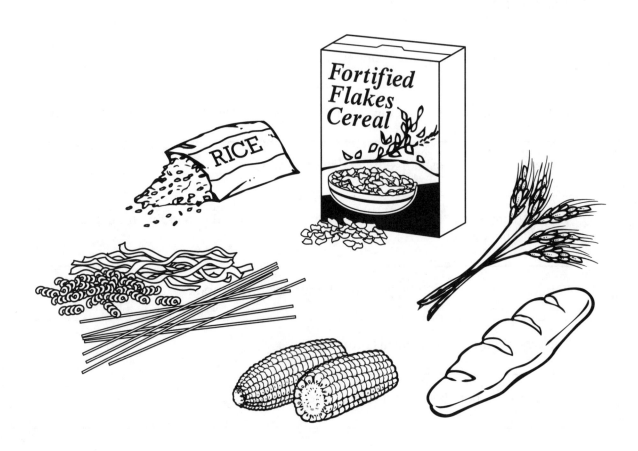

Section 17-2

Activity

Preparing Grains and Grain Products

Viewers Write In

Directions: Imagine that you are the host of a 30-minute weekly television show called Cooking with Chris. After you did an episode in the series titled "Great Grains," you received the following letters from viewers. Write a reply to each letter in the space provided.

1. Dear Chris,
   No matter how much I stir, my rice always turns out sticky. What can I do?

   Ben

   Dear Sticky,

   _____

   _____

   Chris

2. Dear Chris,
   I decided to serve millet for a change of pace. I did exactly what I do when I cook rice, but the grain came out hard as little pebbles. Any thoughts?

   Marcus

   Dear Millie,

   _____

   _____

   Chris

3. Dear Chris,
   I have a problem when I fix spaghetti. I rinse the cooked pasta under running water the way you're supposed to, but it always gets cold. Is there a better way?

   Krystin

   Dear Noodles,

   _____

   _____

   Chris

4. Dear Chris,
   I need to cut down on sugars. I am used to adding sugar to many foods, including breakfast cereals. I don't like plain cereal. Do you have any ideas?

   Belinda

   Dear Sweet,

   _____

   _____

   Chris

Activity

Diner

Directions: Although health experts over the past several years have advised increasing your intake of legumes, these foods have long been a staple in this culture. See for yourself by checking out part of this old diner menu. Use the menu to answer the questions that follow.

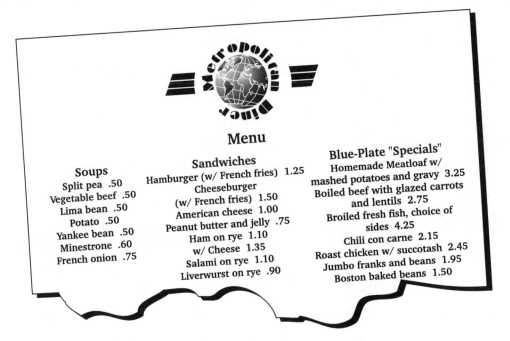

Menu

Soups
Split pea .50
Vegetable beef .50
Lima bean .50
Potato .50
Yankee bean .50
Minestrone .60
French onion .75

Sandwiches
Hamburger (w/ French fries) 1.25
Cheeseburger
(w/ French fries) 1.50
American cheese 1.00
Peanut butter and jelly .75
Ham on rye 1.10
w/ Cheese 1.35
Salami on rye 1.10
Liverwurst on rye .90

Blue-Plate "Specials"
Homemade Meatloaf w/
mashed potatoes and gravy 3.25
Boiled beef with glazed carrots
and lentils 2.75
Broiled fresh fish, choice of
sides 4.25
Chili con carne 2.15
Roast chicken w/ succotash 2.45
Jumbo franks and beans 1.95
Boston baked beans 1.50

1. Which soups on the menu feature legumes in one form or another?

   _____

   _____

2. Which blue plate specials include legumes as part of the meal?

   _____

   _____

3. Are legumes featured at all among the sandwiches? Explain your answer.

   _____

4. Select a soup-and-sandwich lunch from the menu that is meatless but that still offers a serving of protein.

   _____

5. Is it possible to construct a soup-and-sandwich lunch that is meatless and that provides all the essential amino acids? Explain.

   _____

   _____

Chapter 18

Study Guide

Dairy Foods and Eggs

Directions: As you read Chapter 18, answer the following questions. Later you can use this study guide to review chapter information.

Section 18-1   Choosing Dairy Foods

1. Name four nutrients found in milk.

_____

_____

_____

2. What occurs when milk is homogenized? Why is this done?

_____

_____

3. How does yogurt compare nutritionally with milk?

_____

_____

4. What is the difference between ripened and unripened cheese?

_____

_____

_____

5. Identify two ways that butter may be stored and tell how long the butter can be stored each way.

_____

_____

Section 18-2 Preparing Dairy Foods

6. When cooking with milk, how can you keep it from scorching?

_____

_____

7. Explain how to scald milk.

_____

_____

(Continued on next page)

8. How can you reduce the fat in recipes with cheese?

_____

_____

Section 18-3   Egg Basics

9. What limit do nutrition experts recommend with regard to eating eggs? On eating egg whites?

_____

_____

10. How do grade AA eggs compare with grade B eggs in appearance and nutrition?

_____

_____

_____

11. How is egg size determined?

_____

_____

12. Give two tips for choosing eggs in the supermarket.

_____

_____

_____

13. Explain how to move the egg mixture in a skillet when making scrambled eggs.

_____

_____

_____

_____

Section 18-4   Using Eggs in Recipes

14. Describe two functions of eggs in recipes.

_____

_____

15. What is a quiche?

_____

_____

(Continued on next page)

Chapter 18 Study Guide (continued)

16. How are custards baked when prepared in individual cups? What is the reason for this?

_____

_____

_____

17. What is a meringue?

_____

_____

18. Briefly describe the steps in making a meringue.

_____

_____

_____

_____

19. What happens to egg whites if they are overbeaten?

_____

_____

_____

20. Identify two types of meringues and tell how they are used.

_____

_____

_____

Activity

The Case for Dairy

Directions: Your local dairy council is very concerned. A group that calls itself "People Against Dairy" (PAD) has been spreading dangerous rumors about dairy products. The worst part is, the general public is agreeing with PAD! If this trend continues, two problems will occur. First, the general public may not get enough calcium and vitamin D, and second, the decline in dairy sales may force local dairies to lay off almost half of their workers. Since many of this town's citizens work for dairies, the town's economy is at stake. The dairy council has hired you to answer the rumors point by point in the local newspaper. Make the case for dairy products as strong as you can.

PAD's Statements	Your Statements for Dairy Products
1 Milk is very fattening.	_____ _____
2. Milk contains enzymes and microorganisms that cause it to spoil quickly.	_____ _____ _____
3. Milk must be stored in the refrigerator and thus should not be packed in school lunches.	_____ _____ _____ _____ _____
4. Most cheeses get hard when they are stored in the refrigerator, which makes them a poor food value.	_____ _____
5. All frozen dairy products are full of fat.	_____ _____ _____ _____
6. Ice cream picks up an odor when stored at home in the freezer.	_____ _____

Activity

A Happy Ending

Directions: Read the story about Vita's terrible day. Then use your knowledge of dairy foods to rewrite the story so that it has a happy ending. You cannot change the foods she serves, but you can change her actions and food preparation techniques.

Vita was running late. Her guests had already arrived when she finally started lunch. She decided to make a warm yogurt dip to occupy her guests while she cooked lunch. She combined plain yogurt with chopped broccoli, herbs, and spices, and put it in a pan on the stove to heat. While it was warming, she chopped vegetables for her homemade cream of vegetable soup. When she checked on the yogurt, she discovered that it had separated! The dip was a mess! No chance of serving that to guests!

Now she was in even more of a hurry, so she decided to cook the soup over high heat. She dumped the milk and vegetables in the pan all at once to save time. As the mixture warmed up, Vita noticed a skin forming. She carefully removed it with a spoon and went to dump it in the trash. When she returned to the stove, however, she found that the milk had begun to curdle. Vita sighed, quickly turned down the heat, and stirred vigorously, but the damage was done. The soup looked disgusting! She had to serve it anyway because she didn't have anything else to fix. Her guests sipped at their soup politely, but no one finished it.

Your Version of Vita's Day:

_____

_____

_____

_____

_____

_____

_____

_____

_____

_____

_____

_____

_____

_____

_____

_____

Activity

Scrambled Eggs

Directions: The customers at Rudy's restaurant are out of luck this morning. The cook handling the breakfast shift is new at the job and doesn't understand the servers' shorthand expressions. To make matters worse, he lacks experience in preparing eggs. Read each of the descriptions that follow. Using the glossary below, along with information from the textbook, identify (1) the procedure the cook should have followed to prepare the dish in question, and (2) the errors he made in handling eggs. The first one has been partly done for you.

Glossary of Servers' Expressions
Adam and Eve on a raft: Two poached eggs on toast
Make 'em smile: Eggs fried sunny-side up
Mix 'em up but just a little: Eggs scrambled soft
Over easy: Fried eggs, cooked briefly on the second side
Shirley: Baked (shirred) eggs
Speak softly, twice: Two soft-cooked eggs

1. When the server called out "Speak softly, twice!" the cook sprayed cooking oil onto the smoking-hot griddle, and then broke two eggs onto the griddle. After about 12 minutes, he scraped the eggs from the griddle to a plate and placed the plate in the waiting area to be picked up by the server.

   Procedure the cook should have followed: _____
   _____
   _____
   _____

   Error(s) in handling eggs: <u>When frying eggs, which is what the cook evidently thought</u>
   <u>he was supposed to do, you should break one egg at a time into a small bowl; they</u>
   <u>should be cooked over low heat, and only for a short time.</u>

2. When the cook heard an order for "Adam and Eve on a raft," he assumed that it meant ham and cheese omelet. He pan-fried bits of ham in a nonstick skillet. As it was cooking, he broke two eggs into a dish and beat them. When the ham was browned, he added the eggs and some cheese. He slid the finished omelet onto a plate.

   Procedure the cook should have followed: _____
   _____
   _____
   _____

(Continued on next page)

Section 18-3 Activity (continued)

Error(s) in handling eggs: _____

_____

_____

3. The server had just finished preparing a stack of pancakes, when he heard the words "Mix 'em up but just a little." Corned beef hash? he wondered. Assuming that this was what the order was for, he took a couple of eggs from the refrigerator and lowered them into a potful of cold water to poach. Then he started flipping through a cookbook to see if he could locate a recipe for corned beef hash.

Procedure the cook should have followed: _____

_____

_____

_____

Error(s) in handling eggs: _____

_____

_____

4. The server entered the kitchen with an order of "Over easy," which a customer had returned because the eggs were rubbery. "Give me a new order pronto," the server said. Reasoning that maybe the first attempt didn't work because he had left them in the oven too long, the cook decided to try his luck with the microwave. He broke a couple of eggs into a small bowl, and then transferred them to a baking dish. He popped them in the microwave, and set the timer for 40 seconds.

Procedure the cook should have followed: _____

_____

_____

_____

Error(s) in handling eggs: _____

_____

_____

_____

Activity

Missing Parts

Directions: Kerry finally talked his friend Quaranda into writing out the recipe for her delicious lime meringue pie. However, when Kerry read the recipe, he was dismayed to find that she had left a lot to his imagination. Read the recipe Quaranda wrote for her friend, and decide what information is missing. Then use your knowledge of cooking with eggs to rewrite the recipe so that even a beginning cook could follow it. Refer to your textbook if you need help.

Lime Meringue Pie

8-inch (commercial) pie shell

1 cup sugar

⅓ cup cornstarch

1 cup water

2 egg yolks, slightly beaten

1 tsp. grated lime peel

¼ cup lime juice

2 drops green food color

meringue

Bake pie shell according to package directions. Heat oven to 400° F. Place sugar and cornstarch in 1½-quart saucepan and stir in water gradually. Cook over medium heat, stirring constantly until it boils. Stir half the hot mixture gradually into the egg yolks. Blend into mixture in saucepan. Boil and stir 1 minute. Remove from heat. Stir in remaining ingredients. Pour into pie shell. Spread meringue carefully over pie filling to edge of crust. Bake about 10 minutes. Cool.

Lime Meringue Pie

_____
_____
_____
_____
_____
_____
_____
_____
_____
_____

	Chapter 19
Study Guide	**Meat, Poultry, Fish, and Shellfish**

Directions: As you read Chapter 19, answer the following questions. Later you can use this study guide to review chapter information.

Section 19-1   Looking at Meat, Poultry, Fish, and Shellfish

1. What is a cut?

   _____

   _____

2. How do meat, poultry, and fish muscles compare in cholesterol content?

   _____

   _____

3. What is marbling?

   _____

   _____

4. Identify two factors affecting the thickness of muscle fibers.

   _____

   _____

5. Why are all fish and shellfish naturally tender?

   _____

   _____

Section 19-2   Meat Selection and Storage

6. What does the price label on a meat package tell you about the meat?

   _____

   _____

7. Tell what variety meats are, and give four examples.

   _____

   _____

8. Explain the difference between inspection and grading.

   _____

   _____

(Continued on next page)

Chapter 19 Study Guide (continued)

9. Identify one advantage and one disadvantage of processed meats.

_____

_____

_____

Section 19-3 Poultry Selection and Storage

10. What does the term broiler-fryer on a package of chicken indicate? The term capon?

_____

_____

_____

11. What changes might be needed in a recipe when ground poultry is substituted for ground beef?

_____

_____

12. List three organs that might be found in a package of giblets.

_____

_____

13. What is the most common grade of poultry? What does it indicate?

_____

_____

Section 19-4 Fish and Shellfish Selection and Storage

14. What can you do if you don't have the specific type of fish recommended in a recipe?

_____

_____

15. Give three examples of processed fish.

_____

_____

_____

16. What do the letters HACCP stand for? What is HACCP?

_____

_____

_____

(Continued on next page)

Section 19-5 Preparing Meat, Poultry, Fish, and Shellfish

17. Why are moist heat cooking methods good choices for preparing less tender cuts?

_____

_____

18. What is a marinade? What can marinating do for meat?

_____

_____

19. Identify the safest test for doneness in cuts of meat and poultry.

_____

_____

_____

20. Give three tips for browning light-colored cuts cooked in a microwave oven.

_____

_____

_____

Activity

Act One

Directions: Below is a scene from a play in which a family gathers for dinner. Read the scene, and answer the questions.

[The doorbell rings. Cousin Ciel and her husband. Roy, enter.]

Ciel:	Sorry we're late, Aunt Rae. [*Kisses her aunt on the cheek.*] Traffic was awful.
Aunt Rae:	No problem, dear. Come in! Come in and sit down. We're just getting started.
Roy:	[sniffing] Say, Aunt Rae—what is that smell? Is something burning in the kitchen?
Aunt Rae:	Roy, you're such a kidder! That's tonight's dinner—baked scrod.
Uncle Arthur:	Scrod? I don't think I've ever tasted scrod. What kind of meat is that?
Aunt Rae:	It isn't any kind of meat, Arthur. It's fish. [*Family exchanges glances.*]
Uncle Arthur:	Fish! What kind of meal is fish? You've been hosting family dinners for the past 25 years, Rae. You always served braised pot roast at these get-togethers.
Cousin Pete:	Actually, one year she served boiled corned beef and cabbage, Uncle Arthur.
Aunt Rose:	I seem to recall a time when you served us stewed chicken, Rae.
Uncle Arthur:	Corned beef, stewed chicken . . . whatever! The point is, Rae, you've always served us meat—something you can sink your teeth into!
Granny:	[*optimistically*]: Arthur, settle down, dear. Perhaps you're jumping to conclusions. Maybe Rae's intention is to serve us the—uh . . . scrod is it?—as a first course.
Aunt Rae:	No, scrod is tonight's dinner. [*She heads to the kitchen.*]
Uncle Arthur:	I still say, what kind of a meal is fish?
Cousin Pete:	Isn't fish supposed to be brain food?
Roy:	I hear it's good for you.
Uncle Arthur:	Good food, brain food—who cares! Give me a plate full of meat any time!
	[CURTAIN]

1. Which type of meat do you think is eaten most often at the family gatherings—meat with thin or thick muscle fibers? Explain your answer.

   _____

   _____

2. If the meals traditionally eaten at Rae's home were compared with recommendations in the Dietary Guidelines for Americans, how do you think they would shape up nutritionally?

   _____

   _____

3. How does this meal compare with family traditions you've experienced or read about in works of fiction? What does it reveal about Americans' eating plans in the past?

   _____

   _____

Name _____ Date _____ Class _____

Look to the Label

Directions: Below are several meat labels. Use these, plus the information in the textbook, to answer the questions that follow.

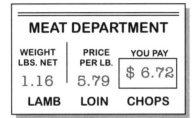

MEAT DEPARTMENT

WEIGHT LBS. NET	PRICE PER LB.	YOU PAY
1.16	5.79	$ 6.72

LAMB   LOIN   CHOPS

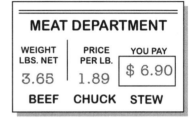

MEAT DEPARTMENT

WEIGHT LBS. NET	PRICE PER LB.	YOU PAY
3.65	1.89	$ 6.90

BEEF   CHUCK   STEW

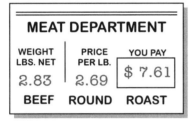

MEAT DEPARTMENT

WEIGHT LBS. NET	PRICE PER LB.	YOU PAY
2.83	2.69	$ 7.61

BEEF   ROUND   ROAST

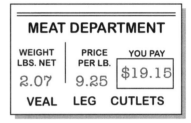

MEAT DEPARTMENT

WEIGHT LBS. NET	PRICE PER LB.	YOU PAY
2.07	9.25	$19.15

VEAL   LEG   CUTLETS

1. Which of these meats is likely to have the heartiest flavor? The mildest?

_____

2. Where on each label does the wholesale cut appear? Where does the retail cut appear?

_____

_____

3. Which of these packages of meat would you plan to cook by moist heat? How would you pre-pare the cuts in the remaining packages? Explain your answers.

_____

_____

_____

4. Which of the cuts would you look for to have a light pink color? A bright red color? Little or no fat?

_____

_____

5. Which of the cuts shown would most likely have a T-shaped bone? Which of the cuts would you expect to have no bone at all? Explain your answers.

_____

_____

_____

Activity

Poultry Meets Its Match

Directions: Read each description of a person's planned meal or favorite recipe. Recommend a type of poultry (being as specific as possible) that will meet that person's needs. Explain your recommendation.

1. Shannon is going to make burgers tonight, but she's worried about the high saturated fat and cholesterol in beef.

   Recommendation: _____

   _____

2. Jerrod is thinking about making his favorite chicken-vegetable soup, but he doesn't have much money to spend on groceries this week.

   Recommendation: _____

   _____

3. Ginny's whole family will be in town next week for a family reunion. She's expecting about 20 people.

   Recommendation: _____

   _____

4. Vance is hungry for hot dogs, but his doctor has told him to stay away from beef and pork products for a while.

   Recommendation: _____

   _____

5. Rich is planning a formal dinner for four. He wants each plate to have its own broiled "bird."

   Recommendation: _____

   _____

6. Everett likes dark meat, but chicken and turkey aren't quite flavorful enough for his taste.

   Recommendation: _____

   _____

Activity

Fish and Shellfish Selection and Storage

Something Fishy

Directions: You are hosting a TV show titled Speak Your Piece. Viewers are able to call in and ask questions or voice concerns. This week's topic is fish. Answer each caller using information from the textbook.

Caller 1: I keep hearing in the news that you should eat more fish. My question is this: Is fish safe to eat? I recently saw a segment on the news about people getting really sick from eating fish.

Your reply: _____

_____

_____

_____

Caller 2: I was in a restaurant recently and saw a fish preparation described as pan-dressed. What exactly does that mean?

Your reply: _____

_____

_____

_____

Caller 3: Help! I'm planning a dinner party for the weekend, and everything is in place—the flowers, the food—everything except the main course. I was planning on making a special salmon with dill sauce, but when I went to the fish store this morning, the manager told me she would not have salmon until Monday. Do you have any suggestions?

Your reply: _____

_____

_____

_____

Caller 4: Can you tell me the difference between crayfish, crawfish, and crawdads? Also, how are they related to lobster?

Your reply: _____

_____

_____

_____

Activity

"Tough Luck" on Teaberry Lane

Directions: It's Saturday, and everyone on Teaberry Lane is dining in. Based on the cuts of meat and cooking methods they have chosen, some families will have tender, delicious meats while others will have "tough luck"! Read the situations. Write "tender" or "tough luck" in each blank.

1. Jenny Templeton roasted a blade roast for her apartment-mates.

   _____

2. Tommy Norton broiled lamb loin chops on his gas grill.

   _____

3. Libby Edgars pan-broiled ground beef patties for her famous double-decker burgers.

   _____

4. Lucas Andrews roasted a stewing hen and made stuffing for his three guests.

   _____

5. Tosha Thomas salted the pork roast before she cooked it.

   _____

6. Terrance Lowry marinated the rib-eye steaks for four hours before cooking them on the charcoal grill.

   _____

7. Lydia Taylor cooked the pork chops in the microwave until they reached an internal temperature of 190°F.

   _____

8. Lester Richardson braised flank steaks for his weekend guests.

   _____

Study Guide

Directions: As you read Chapter 20, answer the following questions. Later you can use this study guide to review chapter information.

Section 20-1   Sandwiches, Snacks, and Packed Lunches

1. Give three suggestions for sandwich fillings.

_____

_____

_____

2. Explain how to make a club sandwich.

_____

_____

_____

3. Describe three guidelines that should be followed when assembling a packed lunch.

_____

_____

_____

_____

Section 20-2 Salads and Dressings

4. What is an emulsion?

_____

_____

5. Explain how to core and clean iceberg lettuce.

_____

_____

_____

_____

6. What is a salad base? What is a salad body?

_____

_____

7. What salad mixtures can be used for molded salads?

_____

(Continued on next page)

Section 20-3 Soups and Sauces

8. What is a bouillon? By what other name is it known?

_____

_____

9. What is a purée? What are the advantages of purées over cream soups?

_____

_____

_____

10. What is a roux?

_____

_____

11. How does pan gravy differ from white sauce?

_____

_____

Section 20-4 Casseroles and Other Combinations

12. How long does it take a stew to cook on top of the range? In a microwave oven? In a slow cooker?

_____

_____

_____

13. Describe the steps in braising meat or poultry.

_____

_____

_____

_____

_____

14. What is the secret to a successful stir-fry?

_____

_____

15. What is an extender? What is a binder?

_____

_____

Activity

Pack a Snack

Directions: Pack two healthful snacks that are appropriate for each of the following situations. List foods inside each plastic zip-up bag. You may not use any food more than once.

1. A snack to take on a bike ride.

2. A snack to serve friends who are coming over to watch a movie.

3. A snack for a three-hour flight.

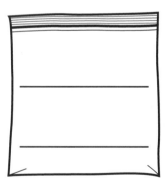

4. A snack for the 15-minute break between exams.

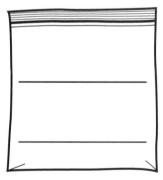

5. A snack for an afternoon by the pool.

6. A midnight snack to follow an evening of sledding.

Activity

Tips from Tiffany

Directions: Tiffany's salad-making abilities are well known in the little town of Drew's Point. Tiffany answers questions and helps people with their salad problems in her weekly column, "Tips from Tiffany." However, Tiffany is on vacation this week, and you are filling in. Answer each of the letters below.

Dear Tiffany:
I love salads and
does my family.
problem is that
get home f

1. Dear Tiffany,
   Last night I served a chef's salad as an appetizer, followed by a roast of lamb and all the trimmings. My guests ate the salad, but then they didn't eat much of the rest of the meal. What did I do wrong?

   Hapless Host

   Dear Hapless,

   _____

   _____

   _____

   _____

   _____

2. Dear Tiffany,
   My coleslaw always makes a big hit at my company's annual picnic. In fact, friends in the office recently asked if I planned to bring it again this year. I've been reading, however, about all the health risks when you eat raw eggs—which is what I use in the dill mayonnaise dressing for the dish. I don't want to let everyone down. Any ideas?

   Harried Harriet

   Dear Harried,

   _____

   _____

   _____

   _____

   _____

(Continued on next page)

3. Dear Tiffany,

   I love salads, and so does my family. The problem is that we all get home for dinner at different times these days, with the kids' after-school activities and my wife's and my own work schedules. What this means is that by the time the last person sits down at the table for dinner, the salad is pretty limp. We can't and don't want to change our lifestyles. What can we change?

   Dad with a Dilemma

Dear Dad,

_____

_____

_____

_____

_____

4. Dear Tiffany,

   I had the most delicious creamy salad dressing at a restaurant recently. When I raved about it to the waiter, he came back with a copy of the recipe, courtesy of the chef. I'd like to make it, but it's so rich and fattening. It's made with mayonnaise, sour cream, mustard, and (the best part!) crushed black peppercorns. Do you know of a dressing like this one that isn't so high in calories or fat?

   Wishful Wanda

Dear Wanda,

_____

_____

_____

_____

_____

Activity

The Saucier's Apprentice

Directions: Shanda has just graduated from cooking school and landed her first job. She will be assisting the saucier—French for "sauce chef"—in an exclusive hotel restaurant. The saucier, Jacqueline, has left a list of preparatory tasks for Shanda to do. First, check the items on hand (in the box below), and make a shopping list of ingredients you will need to complete the tasks. (You may assume that anything not in the pantry needs to be purchased.) Next, decide the order in which you will perform the tasks, and write an explanation of your decision.

Shanda:
Please prepare a pot
of each of the following
for this evening's dinner
shift:
✓ Cream of leek soup
✓ Consommé
✓ Beef stock
✓ Turnip purée
✓ White sauce
✓ Chicken stock
Thank you,

Jacqueline

Kitchen Pantry/Refrigerator

◆ Onions

◆ Carrots

◆ Potatoes

◆ Turnips

◆ Chicken

◆ All-purpose flour

◆ Butter

◆ Assorted seasonings

Ingredients you will need to buy:

_____

_____

_____

Order in which you will perform the tasks:

_____

_____

_____

Explanation for your decision:

_____

_____

_____

_____

Activity

Creative Combos

Directions: Review cookbooks or other recipe sources to find recipes for casseroles and other combination dishes. Adapt, combine, and substitute ingredients to create original recipes for a casserole, pizza, stew, and stir-fry. Select one recipe to test in the foods lab or at home. Evaluate your results in the space provided.

Casserole

_____
_____
_____
_____
_____
_____
_____
_____
_____
_____

Pizza

_____
_____
_____
_____
_____
_____
_____
_____
_____

(Continued on next page)

Stew

_____
_____
_____
_____
_____
_____
_____
_____
_____
_____
_____

Stir-Fry

_____
_____
_____
_____
_____
_____
_____
_____
_____
_____
_____

Recipe selected for testing: _____

_____

Evaluation of results: _____

_____

16. Why are foam cakes baked in ungreased pans?

_____

_____

17. What is the main difference between cookies and cakes? What is the result of this difference?

_____

_____

18. What should you remember when placing drop cookies on a cookie sheet?

_____

_____

19. Why should you let cookie sheets cool before baking more cookies?

_____

_____

20. When making piecrust, what is the procedure for transferring the rolled pastry dough circle from a floured surface and fit it into a pie pan?

_____

_____

Activity

Baker's Dozen

Directions: The term baker's dozen refers to not 12 items, as in a standard dozen, but 13. It traces its origins to the sixteenth century, when the phrase was used as a code among bakers in the courts of kings. Whenever these early artisans received orders to bake a dozen cakes for a banquet or feast, they would routinely requisition enough ingredients to make a "baker's dozen"—keeping the extra cake for themselves and their families. Below are a "baker's half dozen"—seven—tips that might have appeared in a recipe book for baking in the late Middle Ages. Read each tip, and identify it as either fact or fancy in terms of the current state of food science. If it is fancy, write the correct explanation in the space provided.

Tip 1. One ought to take great care, when crafting a baked good that is to rise up high in the pan, to include a liquid of some kind. Once placed in the hearth, this same liquid—be it milk of cows, soured milk [buttermilk], or water from the well—will alone yield the desired outcome. Omit the liquid, and a flat pancake shall be the result no matter what else is used in the Receipt [recipe].

Fact or fancy: _____

Corrected information: _____

_____

_____

Tip 2. When the whole of the grain alone be used in bakery [baked goods], a much weightier product be your lot [the result].

Fact or fancy: _____

Corrected information: _____

_____

_____

Tip 3. One may add spice (viz., Clove, Nut Meg, All Spice) to bakery for sweetness. One may add as well the cane of the Sugar plant, be it in syrup or powdered form; this too shall sweeten the product, though no other known purpose be served by its addition.

Fact or fancy: _____

Corrected information: _____

_____

_____

(Continued on next page)

Section 21-1 Activity (continued)

Tip 4. Fat, such as lard or dairy butter, lends bakery a rich flavour and ensures, moreover, that a cake be tender. One need use only the tiniest trace to derive these benefits.

Fact or fancy: _____

Corrected information: _____

_____

_____

Tip 5. It has been noted elsewhere—and bears repetition herein—that when thickened cream or custard be used to fill cakes or other sweet bakery, such end products must be consumed at once or stored without in the chill winter air; elsewise, the product may turn rank and most unappetising.

Fact or fancy: _____

Corrected information: _____

_____

_____

Tip 6. If bakery is to please the King, great pains need be taken to use the best butter and eggs, and to mix together such ingredients with extreme care. The order of combination of the ingredients makes little difference whatsoever, so long as they be of the finest quality.

Fact or fancy: _____

Corrected information: _____

_____

_____

Tip 7. Upon removing bread from the hearth, turn it out upon a grate, lest the loaf turn damp from direct placement upon the table top or baker's bench.

Fact or fancy: _____

Corrected information: _____

_____

_____

Activity

Bread Alert

Directions: Read the situations involving preparation of quick breads. For each situation that shows an incorrect procedure or outcome, draw a "Bread Alert" flag in the box and explain the problem in the space provided. If the procedure or outcome is correct, leave the box blank. The first situation has already been done for you.

1. Ina's muffin batter contained lots of floury spots as she spooned it into the baking cups.
   It should have only a few floury spots.

2. Mary's muffin batter was somewhat lumpy.

3. Sharon substituted 1½ cups bran for 1½ cups flour to add fiber to her muffins.

4. Mike sifted together the dry ingredients for muffins.

5. Thad lined the loaf pan with waxed paper before spooning in the batter.

6. The top of the loaf of banana bread cracked during baking.

7. Stu filled the muffin cups $7/8$ full.

8. Lori spooned the cranberry bread batter into the ungreased loaf pan.

Activity

Say "Yes" to Yeast Breads

Directions: Read the following statements about steps in making yeast breaks. Check "Yes" for statements that are correct; check "No" for those that are not correct. Use the space provided to explain why the "No" statements are incorrect.

YES   **NO**

_____   _____   1. The microwave oven is useful in several steps of yeast bread making.

_____

_____   _____   2. The only way to knead yeast dough is with your hands.

_____

_____   _____   3. Yeast bread contains baking powder.

_____

_____   _____   4. Salt in yeast bread controls the action of the yeast.

_____

_____   _____   5. Bread flour is the only suitable flour for making yeast bread.

_____

_____   _____   6. Ingredients for yeast bread should be at room temperature.

_____

_____   _____   7. Very hot liquids are necessary to activate yeast.

_____

_____   _____   8. Knead yeast dough until it becomes a smooth, dull ball.

_____

(Continued on next page)

YES   **NO**

_____   _____   9. Adding too much extra flour to yeast dough will make the bread tough.

_____

_____   _____   10. Some types of flour absorb more liquid than others.

_____

_____   _____   11. Something is wrong with your yeast dough if air bubbles form while you knead it.

_____

_____   _____   12. Allow yeast dough to rise in a well-oiled bowl.

_____

_____   _____   13. Do not cover the dough while it is rising.

_____

_____   _____   14. Punch the dough down with your fist after the first rising.

_____

_____   _____   15. If dough is ready for shaping, it will spring back when touched.

_____

_____   _____   16. Yeast dough should never be refrigerated before you shape it.

_____

_____   _____   17. Yeast loaves cut more easily just after they are removed from the pans.

_____

Activity

Alike and Different

Directions: In some ways, cakes, cookies, and pies each have unique features. At the same time, these baked delicacies share a number of common traits. The statements below and on the next page consist of both unique and shared features. Read each statement; then write the letter that precedes it in one or more of the boxes beneath the appropriate drawing(s).

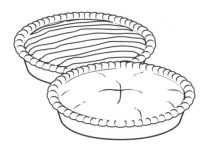

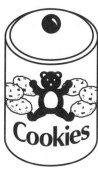

A. These treats are traditionally high in fat, sugar, and calories.

B. There are two basic types of these—shortened and foam.

C. These are best stored in a covered container, with waxed paper between layers to keep them from sticking together.

D. The dough for these is rolled out on a lightly floured surface.

E. These are baked on flat pans with only one edge.

F. These baked delicacies take their name from a Dutch word meaning "little cakes."

G. You can test these for doneness by lightly touching the top and checking to see whether it springs back.

(Continued on next page)

H. These can be filled with a sweet or savory mixture.

I. For added eye appeal, use a fork to make indentations along the edge of these.

J. During baking, the dough spreads out.

K. It is a good idea to line the bottom of the pan with parchment paper so that these can be removed easily after they have finished baking.

L. The basic ingredients for the dough for these is flour, fat, salt, and water.

M. These can be baked in a wide variety of shapes and sizes.

N. The bar variety of these are done baking when they pull away slightly from the sides of the pan.

O. These may contain a fruit, custard, or cream filling, and are generally served as a dessert.

	Chapter 22
# Study Guide	**Foods of the World**

Directions: As you read Chapter 22, answer the following questions. Later you can use this study guide to review chapter information.

Section 22-1   Latin America

1. What is the staple grain in much of Latin America?

   _____

   _____

2. What is masa?

   _____

   _____

3. Compare the Costa Rican preparation of chayote with that of the Dominican Republic.

   _____

   _____

   _____

4. Identify three fruits and two vegetables that are basic to Caribbean cooking.

   _____

   _____

   _____

5. Identify one of Argentina's main food products and describe one way it is often served.

   _____

   _____

Section 22-2   Africa and the Middle East

6. Identify three ways yams are prepared in Africa.

   _____

   _____

   _____

7. Describe a typical African evening meal.

   _____

   _____

   _____

   _____

(Continued on next page)

8. What is couscous? Name two ways in which couscous is served.

_____

_____

_____

9. Name two fruits, two vegetables, and two seasonings associated with Middle Eastern cooking.

_____

_____

_____

10. What legume is featured in falafel? In what other Israeli dish is it featured?

_____

_____

_____

Section 22-3 Europe

11. Identify three dishes often served for lunch or dinner in Great Britain.

_____

_____

12. Identify and describe two examples of cuisine bourgeoise.

_____

_____

_____

_____

_____

13. What is fruksoppa? Where is it eaten? How is it made?

_____

14. For what dish are the Hungarian people most famous? What ingredients does this dish contain?

_____

_____

Section 22-4 Asia and the Pacific

15. List four staples of the traditional Japanese diet.

_____

_____

16. What are the two main parts of a typical Korean meal?

_____

_____

(Continued on next page)

17. What seasonings are commonly used with fish and other foods in Vietnam?

_____

_____

18. What are the staple foods of the Philippines? How are they used?

_____

_____

19. Describe two ways in which the cooking of northern and southern India differ.

_____

_____

_____

20. What is Pavlova?

_____

_____

Activity

Lunch Latin American Style

Directions: Foods from Latin America include a wide variety of interesting, flavorful dishes. Write the names of the following foods on the map in the country or region where they are found. Then plan a lunch menu using one or more Latin American foods, and write the menu inside the circle.

carbonada criolla
mariscada
pollo con mole
    poblano

ceviche
feijoada
empanada

frijoles refritos
moros y cristianos

chayote
gazpacho

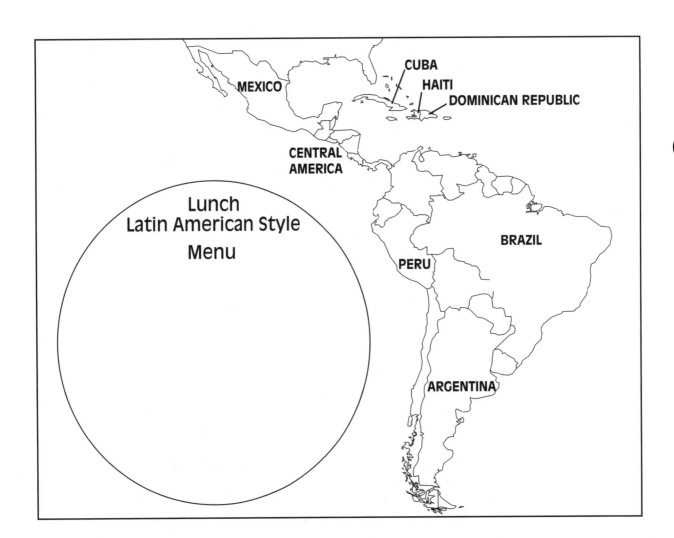

Activity

Foods, Climates, and Cultures

Directions: For each country listed below, identify the general geography and climate (or climates) and describe at least two typical foods eaten there. (This may take some research. You may need to refer to a world atlas or an encyclopedia.)

Morocco
Geography/Climate: _____

_____

_____

Foods: _____

_____

_____

Israel
Geography/Climate: _____

_____

_____

Foods: _____

_____

_____

Ethiopia
Geography/Climate: _____

_____

_____

Foods: _____

_____

_____

Mali
Geography/Climate: _____

_____

Foods: _____

_____

_____

(Continued on next page)

Section 22-2 Activity (continued)

Botswana
Geography/Climate: _____

_____

Foods: _____

_____

_____

Angola
Geography/Climate: _____

_____

Foods: _____

_____

_____

Oman
Geography/Climate: _____

_____

Foods: _____

_____

_____

Activity

ABC's of European Dining

Directions: For each description below and on the next page, identify the food or culinary term beginning with the letter shown. Then describe the food or term.

A _____

1. Italian term for "before the meal."

   Description: _____

   _____

B _____

2. Originally made by the fishermen's wives in the south of France with fish left over from the day's catch.

   Description: _____

C _____

3. A breakfast staple enjoyed in Spain with coffee or hot chocolate.

   Description: _____

D _____

4. An easy and economical way of making a sauce.

   Description: _____

   _____

E _____

5. The name by which Americans know this British teatime staple.

   Description: _____

F _____

6. A direct translation of "fruit soup."

   Description: _____

   _____

G _____

7. Often written phonetically as goulash in our culture.

   Description: _____

   _____

   _____

H _____

8. Literally, "high cooking" in France.

   Description: _____

   _____

   _____

I _____

9. Country where you would be served a contorno after the main course.

   Description: _____

(Continued on next page)

Section 22.3 Activity (continued)

J _____

10. An ingredient of an Austrian dessert that is a cross between a pie and a cake.

   Description: _____

   _____

K _____

11. A Czech dessert that is one of the most famous dishes of that culture.

   Description: _____

   _____

L _____

12. A festive dessert that translates as "Lucia buns."

   Description: _____

   _____

M _____

13. A rib-sticking dish that features Greece's most popular meat.

   Description: _____

   _____

N _____

14. A spice-flavored cake or cookie of German origin that is often shaped like a person in our own culture.

   Description: _____

P _____

15. A dish common in the North of Italy, where it is eaten in place of pasta.

   Description: _____

   _____

Activity

Food and Philosophies File

Directions: This file will help you uncover important facts about foods and philosophies of the people of Asia and the Pacific islands. First, write the correct word on the blanks beneath each description. The numbers beneath the answer blanks correspond to numbers on the file drawers. To check your work, find the drawer that corresponds to the number beneath each blank. The letter you wrote in each blank should be one of the letters on that file drawer.

1. A mixture of vegetables and meat cooked quickly in a wok

   ___ ___ ___ ___ ___ ___ ___ ___
   6   6   4   3   7   1   4   3

2. Used in Korea to add interest and flavor to dishes

   ___ ___ ___ ___ ___ ___ ___
   5   3   1   4   4   2   6

3. A province of central China noted for its use of hot peppers

   ___ ___ ___ ___ ___ ___ ___ ___
   6   7   2   1   3   7   1   4

4. The national dish of the Philippines

   ___ ___ ___ ___ ___
   1   2   5   1   5

5. A pungent fish sauce used as a seasoning in Vietnam

   ___ ___ ___ ___   ___ ___ ___
   4   6   5   1   4   1   4

6. The foundation of virtually all recipes in India

   ___ ___ ___ ___ ___   ___ ___ ___ ___ ___ ___
   3   1   5   1   4   4   1   6   1   4   1

7. A unique Australian dish of meringue, fruit, and cream

   ___ ___ ___ ___ ___ ___ ___
   5   1   6   4   5   6   1

File cabinet drawers:
- ABC — 1
- DEF — 2
- GHIJ — 3
- KLMN — 4
- OPQR — 5
- STUV — 6
- WXYZ — 7

(Continued on next page)

Name _____ Date _____ Class _____

Section 22-4 Activity (continued)

8. A Canton specialty featuring broad noodles stir-fried with strips of meat, onions, and bean sprouts

__ __ __ __   __ __ __
1 3 5 7   2 6 4

9. A popular Thai dish made of noodles, shrimp, peanuts, eggs, and bean sprouts

__ __ __   __ __ __ __
5 1 2   6 3 1 3

10. An Indonesian dish of fried rice surrounded by assorted meats

__ __ __ __ __ __ __ __ __ __
4 1 6 3 3 5 5 2 4 3

11. Dietary guidelines in this country recommend 30 different foods a day

__ __ __ __ __
3 1 5 1 4

12. View of food preparation in China—a _____ of opposites

__ __ __ __ __ __ __
1 1 4 1 4 1 2

13. In Japan, crisp batter-fried vegetables and seafood

__ __ __ __ __ __ __
6 2 4 5 6 5 1

14. Indonesian salad of lettuce, hard-cooked eggs, onions, and bean sprouts, topped with a peanut butter–based dressing

__ __ __ __   __ __ __ __
3 1 2 5   3 1 2 5

15. Food that resembles clams, enjoyed by New Zealanders

__ __ __ __ __ __ __ __
6 5 3 2 5 5 1 6

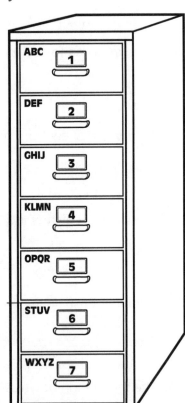

Chapter 23

Study Guide

Foods of the U.S. and Canada

Directions: As you read Chapter 23, answer the following questions. Later you can use this study guide to review chapter information.

Section 23-1 Regional Foods of the East, Midwest, and South

1. Describe two ways in which Native Americans were "early pioneers in food technology."

   _____

   _____

   _____

2. Identify two dishes that early immigrants in the Northeast learned from the Native Americans.

   _____

3. Name three foods that the Pennsylvania Dutch brought to America from Germany.

   _____

   _____

4. In general, on what did Midwestern pioneers rely to flavor their meals?

   _____

5. Identify the staple crop of the South in the eighteenth century and four foods made from it.

   _____

   _____

6. Name two foods with African-American roots, and explain what each one is.

   _____

   _____

   _____

7. In general, how does Creole cooking differ from Cajun cooking?

   _____

   _____

8. What is filé powder? For what was it used?

   _____

Section 23-2 Regional Foods of the West and Canada

9. Describe a typical cowboy meal.

   _____

   _____

(Continued on next page)

10. Describe two Tex-Mex dishes.

_____

_____

_____

_____

11. How was sourdough bread introduced to the Northwest?

_____

_____

12. Identify four cultures that have contributed to Hawaiian cooking.

_____

_____

13. In what part of Canada are râpée pie and colcannon eaten? Describe these dishes.

_____

_____

_____

14. By what name do Canadians call the bacon known in the United States as Canadian bacon? How is this different from streaky bacon?

_____

_____

15. What berry is grown in abundance in British Columbia? What two berries is it a cross between?

_____

_____

Activity

From There to Where?

Directions: Below is a list of "all-American" foods or food phenomena. Write each term in a box with the label of the culture where it arose. Write each term again in the section of the map on the next page to show where in the United States the custom was adopted.

baked beans
Cajun gumbo
clam chowder
coffee klatch
corn bread
corn pone
corned beef and cabbage

filé powder
Hopping John
hush puppies
peach cobbler
pecan pie
scrapple

Native American	**Irish**

Pennsylvania Dutch	**African-American**

French Canadian

(Continued on next page)

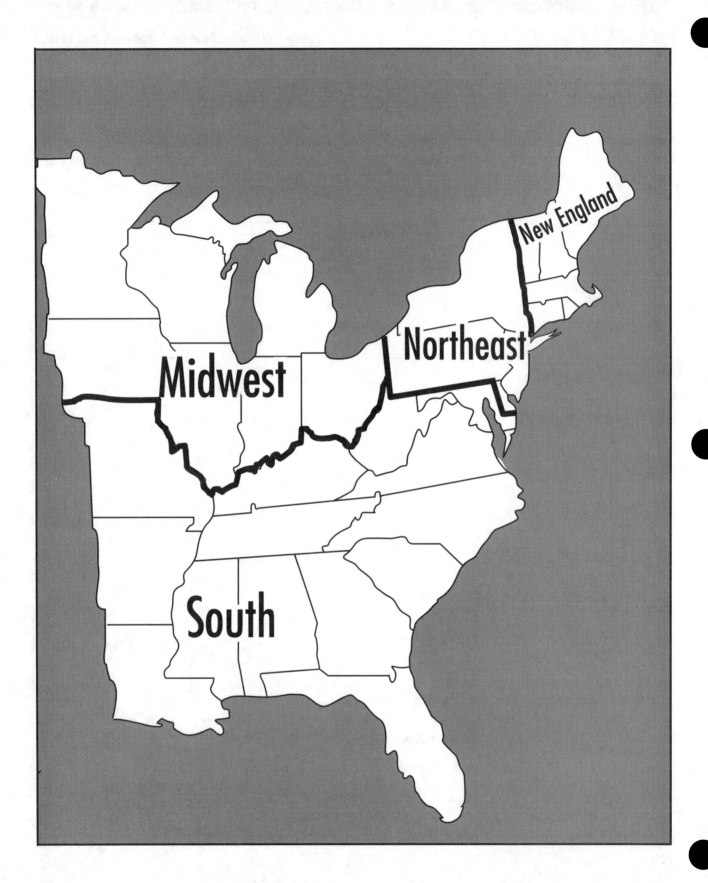

Activity

Roundup of Cooks, Cuisines, and Cultures

Directions: Imagine that this is the nineteenth century. Use the space provided to write a short paragraph about how you would find and prepare foods to feed your family if you lived in each of these regions. Use your textbook and any other references you may need.

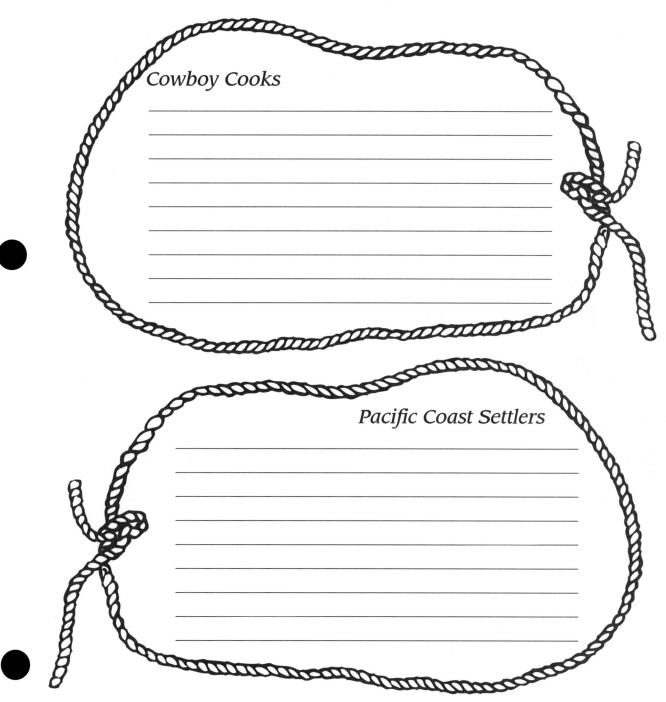

Cowboy Cooks

Pacific Coast Settlers

(Continued on next page)

Island Inhabitants

_____
_____
_____
_____
_____
_____
_____

Canadian Nationalities

_____
_____
_____
_____
_____
_____
_____

Study Guide

Directions: As you read Chapter 24, answer the following questions. Later you can use this study guide to review chapter information,

Section 24-1   Creative Techniques

1. What are herbs?

   _____

   _____

2. What are spices?

   _____

   _____

3. How should herbs and spices be stored?

   _____

   _____

4. What are condiments? Name two examples.

   _____

   _____

   _____

5. What should you remember about size, color, and flavor when garnishing foods?

   _____

   _____

   _____

Section 24-2   Beverages

6. Identify three nutrients in milk.

   _____

   _____

7. What is mulled cider?

   _____

   _____

8. What is instant coffee? How is it prepared?

   _____

   _____

(Continued on next page)

9. How should you clean a coffee carafe and basket? Why?

_____

_____

Section 24-3   Entertaining

10. List four types of information that should be included on an invitation.

_____

_____

11. Give two qualities of an appropriate buffet food.

_____

_____

12. How is the starting point at a reception table indicated?

_____

_____

13. Give four examples of possible food choices for a reception.

_____

_____

Section 24-4   Outdoor Meals

14. What might happen if you allow baked-on grime to accumulate on a grill?

_____

_____

15. Explain how to dispose of burning charcoal properly after grilling.

_____

_____

16. Identify an especially important food safety consideration when serving meals outdoors.

_____

_____

17. Give two tips for using a cooler at the picnic site.

_____

_____

(Continued on next page)

Section 24-5 Preserving Food at Home

18. What is dry-packing?

_____

_____

_____

19. When canning foods, can you change the recipe to decrease the salt or sugar content? Explain.

_____

_____

20. What is meant by processing foods?

_____

_____

Section 24-1

Activity

Creative Techniques

Seasoned Just Right

Directions: In the blanks provided, write the word that best completes each statement. Place one letter in each blank. Then transfer the circled letters to the shakers to reveal the seasoning secret.

1. Herbs are flavorful __ __ __ __ __ (__) and stems of soft, succulent plants that grow in the temperate zone.

2. The three main enemies of herbs and spices are __ __ __ __ (__), air, and heat.

3. __ __ (__) __ __ __ __ __ __ blends are convenient combinations of herbs and spices.

4. A strongly flavored herb that is used heavily in Mexican and Italian cooking is __ (__) __ __ __ __ __.

5. Dried herbs are more __ __ (__) __ __ __ than fresh.

6. Dried ground buds, bark, seeds, stems, or roots of aromatic plants are known as (__) __ __ __ __ __

7. Liquids used to accompany and complement food flavors are known as __ __ __ __ __ (__) __ __ __ __.

8. A sweetly flavored spice that is used with fruit dishes, sweet potatoes, and squash is __ __ __ __ (__) __ __ __ .

9. Cooking in parchment paper, or en __ __ __ __ __ (__) __ __ __ , is a method creative cooks use.

10. A popular condiment for Mexican foods is __ __ (__) __ __.

The seasoning secret is:

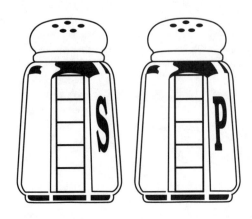

Activity

Beating the Beverage Blues

Directions: Each of the following people has had a disappointing experience with a beverage. On the lines below each person's statement, tell what the person could have done differently to achieve better results.

1. Alexis received an expensive flavored coffee for her birthday. After brewing one carafe, she decided to use it only for special occasions, so she folded the package down, closed it, and put it in a cabinet. When she used it again two months later, the coffee had lost most of its flavor and tasted bitter.

   _____

   _____

   _____

2. Arthur came in feeling hot after his softball game and craved something cold to drink. He had always enjoyed iced tea but had never made it. He prepared hot tea just as he always did at breakfast time and then put ice cubes in it. He didn't think much of it though; it was too watery!

   _____

   _____

   _____

3. As Pierre headed out of the decoration committee meeting for a beverage, he offered to take orders for other members. Zak asked Pierre to bring him back something with fruit juice in it, so he could get one of his daily servings of fruit. When Pierre returned with a can of orange soda that read "10 percent fruit juice" on the label, Zak was disappointed.

   _____

   _____

   _____

4. Ruben enjoys trying new types of tea. Recently, he bought a package of orange cinnamon spice tea. When he got home, he realized that it was loose tea. He made the tea and used cheesecloth to strain out the tea leaves, but it didn't work all that well. The tea was delicious, but some of the tea particles slipped through the cheesecloth into the tea.

   _____

   _____

   _____

Activity

The Party Plan

Directions: Use the form below to plan a party for the occasion of your choice. Follow the appropriate guidelines in your text.

Event/occasion: _____

_____

Check one: _____ Formal _____ Informal

Theme: _____

_____

Menu: _____

_____

_____

_____

_____

_____

_____

Method for Serving: _____

_____

Activities: _____

_____

_____

_____

_____

_____

Decorations: _____

_____

_____

Form of Invitation: _____

_____

_____

Activity

Class Picnic

Directions: The school year is ending, and to celebrate, students in Class 222 are holding a year-end picnic. Read the statements below which describe selected moments of the day. If the description shows good food safety for outdoor meals, write a check mark on the line before it. If the description shows improper safety, place an X on the line and explain what the student should have done.

_____ 1. When fat dripped down from the burgers on the grill, causing flames to shoot up, Al Schenk—who was manning the grill—did his impersonation of the hero in the movie *Flamy Inferno*.

_____ 2. Lori Spellman didn't want her banana cream pie to get crushed, so she placed it at the top of the cooler, with all the soft drink cans underneath.

_____ 3. Brad Richie brought assorted sandwiches and fresh fruit for anyone who wanted them. He kept them in a chilled insulated container.

_____ 4. Vanessa Calendar wanted to serve her famous grilled chicken but didn't want to spend the day over a hot grill. So she partially cooked the seasoned chicken in her microwave oven at home that morning, brought it warm to the picnic, and finished cooking it in time for dinner, after everyone had taken a dip in the lake.

Activity

Worth Preserving

Directions: The following are claims for inventions that currently do not exist but that some day might help people with the task of home preserving. Read each claim and identify the type of home preserving each is designed to facilitate. Note: Some types of preserving may appear more than once.

1. The new Blanch-o-matic can shave valuable time off this home preserving task.

   _____

2. New from Blammo Industries, the space-age "High and Dry" keeps foods at a constant temperature of 90°F (32°C).

   _____

3. No need to guess whether you've left ample room when preserving—thanks to the all-new Headspacer, which takes the guesswork out of home preserving.

   _____

4. You say you want to do a lot of preserving in a little bit of space? Now you can, with Biffmore's Dry-Packer. Great for crowded city apartments.

   _____

5. Are you eager to preserve but frustrated because the kitchen range isn't working? No problem when you have the Zipco Hot-Packer on your side!

   _____

6. Are you fed up with running out of sugar just when you need it most? Never again, with Sugar-Packies! These amazing new quick-dissolving sugar tablets make your home preserving chores a snap.

   _____

7. Make your own beef jerky in seconds with Dehydro, the amazing high-tech way to preserve at home. One 1-milligram tablet of Dehydro makes up to a pound of delicious, tangy jerky.

   _____

Study Guide

Directions: As you read Chapter 25, answer the following questions. Later you can use this study guide to review chapter information.

Section 25-1 Career Opportunities

1. How do employees advance in a career?

2. What types of services are included in the food service industry?

3. What are the educational requirements for a job in the food service industry?

4. What does the field of family and consumer sciences involve?

5. What work is done by food researchers?

6. Identify two types of work done by food scientists.

7. What is a dietitian?

8. What is an entrepreneur?

(Continued on next page)

Chapter 25 Study Guide (continued)

9. Identify three personal qualities of successful entrepreneurs.

_____

_____

Section 25-2   The Successful Worker

10. Why is the ability to learn an important quality in an employee?

_____

_____

_____

11. Identify three qualities of a good resumé.

_____

_____

_____

12. What types of information are you not required to give on a job application?

_____

_____

13. Why is the content and appearance of an application form or resumé so important?

_____

_____

_____

14. Name three documents you may need for employment.

_____

_____

15. If you were fired from your job, how should you handle that fact in your next job interview?

_____

_____

_____

Activity

Where the Jobs Are

Directions: This activity will help you find out where the jobs are in the food and nutrition field. The keys below unlock doors opening on six major career areas. Work on unlocking one door at a time. Identify names from the Job List of three jobs in that career area. Write the letters of those jobs in the left column (labeled "Job"). Then turn the page and find three examples on the List of Examples that illustrate the jobs you identified. Write the number of each example in the right column beside the job it illustrates.

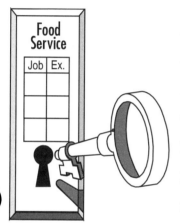

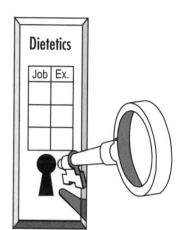

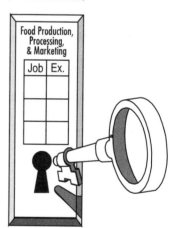

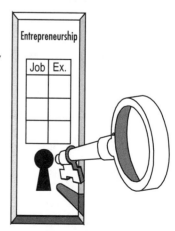

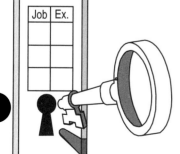

Job List

A. Developing recipes

B. Laboratory science

C. Health maintenance organization

D. Catering

E. Teaching adults through extension

F. Managing a bakery

G. Food delivery service

H. Farming

I. Test kitchen worker

J. Serving food

K. Nutrition consulting service

L. Editor of a consumer magazine

M. Chef of a fine restaurant

N. Product developer for manufacturer

O. Hospital dietitian

P. Consumer advocate for government agency

Q. Managing a supermarket

R. Nursing home nutrition director

(Continued on next page)

List of Examples

1. Carlos finished the management training program and became manager of a large supermarket.

2. George is the head waiter at an Italian restaurant.

3. Jane plans menus for patients in the maternity and pediatric wards.

4. In her county, Fran is in charge of adult courses in food preservation.

5. Ted's income from his wheat crop is quite good this year.

6. Catherine finds the experimental work in the company lab fascinating.

7. Gerald decided to open his own business as a consultant for people with dietary concerns.

8. Reginald found his work with the USDA very satisfying, especially when he was able to offer valuable help to consumers in need.

9. Grace liked the excitement of working at Foodco; she was proud of the new food forms she had helped develop.

10. Julio is the head chef at a hotel resort.

11. Carolyn performs diet analyses at the Health-Pro Organization.

12. Susan enjoys planning and preparing for receptions and formal dinners.

13. Heather plans menus for patients at Shady Lawn Nursing Center.

14. Timothy writes and edits articles for a consumer magazine.

15. Sean plans to take over the family bakery when his father retires.

16. Germaine enjoys testing new recipes and analyzing their nutritional value.

17. Carl's new business offers the first home food delivery service in the city.

18. Cherise's task is to create new recipes to enable the new restaurant to compete with other restaurants in town.

Activity

Express for Success

Directions: Being able to express yourself is an important skill for success in the world of work. Both verbal and nonverbal forms of expression are important. Practice your communication skills by following the instructions in each situation below. You may want to keep a copy of this exercise on file for future reference.

1. How would you answer this interview question: Why should we hire you?

   _____

   _____

   _____

   _____

   _____

   _____

   _____

2. Write an opening sentence for a letter of application.

   _____

   _____

   _____

3. Write a closing sentence for a letter of application.

   _____

   _____

   _____

4. Tell how you would respond to an interviewer who questioned you about your religion.

   _____

   _____

   _____

5. List three people you would choose as references. List their roles or their relationships to you.

   _____

   _____

   _____

(Continued on next page)

Name _____ Date _____ Class _____

Section 25-2 Activity (continued)

6. Would you select the chronological or the functional format for your resumé? Explain your choice.

_____

_____

_____

7. Write one question you would ask an interviewer during your job interview.

_____

_____

_____

8. What would you say on the phone to a personnel director in order to obtain an interview?

_____

_____

_____

9. How would you dress for an interview with a food manufacturing company for a position as lab scientist? Be specific and give reasons for your clothing choices.

_____

_____

_____

10. How would you dress for an interview for a position as a server in a hotel banquet room? Be specific and give reasons for your clothing choices.

_____

_____

_____